FRUIT AND VEGETABLES AS MEDICINE

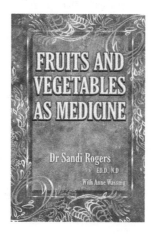

Dr Sandi Rogers ED.D., N.D

With Anne Wassnig

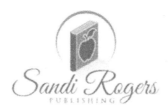

First Published in Australia 1997
Second Edition 2000 15 reprints to 2014
Third edition and upgraded 2015

The information contained in this text is presented as information only, it should not take the place of professional advice. Always consult your wholistically trained health care practitioner.

It is important to also note, that depending on the condition being treated, it may be necessary to use the treatments recommended in conjunction with other medications, as prescribed by your medical practitioner. In this instance you must ascertain the safety of combining foods and pharmaceutical drugs as there maybe an adverse interaction.

The eclectic practitioner will blend treatments that are for you, the person, and not treat a condition. This text is offered as a ready reference for the management of common conditions but not to take the place of a professional consultation.

Countless numbers of people take short cuts and purchase products over the counter thinking they are saving money, yet fail to see they may be spending money on product that is not useful and in fact the only thing that will occur is to make them poorer and develop a very expensive urine.

In this day and age with the plethora of information on the internet, many people self-diagnose and often get it quite wrong. Please find a qualified practitioner who you feel comfortable with and work as a team.

By consulting with a natural medicine consultant you can be assured about safety and receiving the best advice and support, working as a team to achieve your goals.

Phone: 0411047821
Email: sandi@nctm.com.au
Web: www.sandirogers.com.au
Correspondence to: Dr Sandi Rogers
8/32 Ereton Drive, Arundel, QLD, 4214
Sandi Rogers Publishing

National Library of Australia Cataloguing-in-Publication

Creator: Rogers, Dr Sandi,
Title: Fruit and Vegetables as Medicine / Sandi Rogers illustrated by
Laila Savolainen.

ISBN: 9780992569754 (paperback)
ISBN: 9780992569761 (ebook)
Subjects: Fruit—Therapeutic use.
             Vegetables—Therapeutic use.
Dewey Number: 615.321

Book Cover Design: Pickawoowoo, Laila Savolainen
Interior Design: Pickawoowoo Publishing Group

Printed & Channel Distribution
Lightning Source | Ingram (USA/UK/EUROPE/AUS)

Dr Sandi Rogers ED.D., N.D

Sandi is a qualified Educator, Naturopath, Herbalist, Reflexognosist and Public Speaker who draws audiences Internationally. She calls on her experience from running two clinics in Melbourne, Victoria for more than three decades. She now consults on the Gold Coast, Queensland.

She maintains her position as CEO of the National College of Traditional Medicine, respected interstate and international lecturer, public speaker and published author, to deliver this dynamic, exciting updated book.

Enjoy!

Anne Wassnig

Since beginning her career in education Anne has had several publications. She has written education material for the RSPCA, Melbourne Water, and a children's activity book for Healesville Sanctuary. Anne has also written a patient's memoirs for a hospice in Melbourne, and is currently writing for a practitioner of natural therapies.

When beginning this project both Sandi and Anne began by identifying and clarifying the objectives of this book. Through discussion and collaboration, they decided on a format that would provide immediate, easily accessible information regarding fruit and vegetables as medicine. They wanted the reader to be able to gain as little or as much information as they needed or wanted.

Anne then set out to collate and present all the research, provided by Sandi, with the agreed upon format, and in a way that would achieve the objectives. Anne is confident that you will be as happy as she with this book.

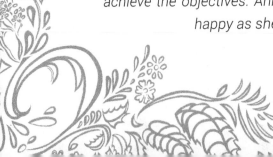

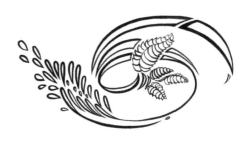

Acknowledgments

I would like to acknowledge all my students and clients who have taught and inspired me so much. I am the student of students, and their input is invaluable to me to assist with my quest for lifelong learning.

Additionally I would like to thank my life partner Ronny for her love, support and stability to guide me through my travels.

To my parents who instilled in me that anything is possible and to my wonderful sister Helen and brother John who are the cream of the crop when it comes to siblings.

To Polly who is with me always.

Dr Sandi Rogers ED.D., N.D

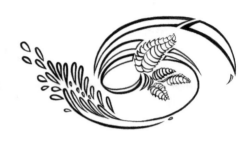

Dedication

I dedicate my efforts to my mother who taught me not to be afraid to be myself and urged me to explore my potential.

Thank you to Roland, Matthew and Sarah for their love, encouragement and support.

Anne Wassnig B.Ed.

  Respectable mainstream groups-
including the National Cancer
Institute and the New York
Academy of Science-agree that
nutrition can play a vital role in the
prevention, treatment, and cure
of a wide variety of ailments .

Earl Mindell, R. Ph. D

  If carrots were used more
extensively as a vegetable,
they would prove of great
benefit to mankind .

Jethro Kloss Author Back to Eden

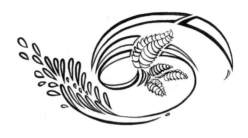

Introduction

Today we are witnessing a great transition in nutritional thinking. The fast foods, with highly processed applications and preservatives, are now being seen to be what they really are, hollow empty substances with little or no nutritional value.

For centuries, food in its most natural state, has been referred to as being the cellular activist for our anatomy. Regeneration takes place with the aid of the foods we consume. This food must in itself live in order for this action to take place. Therefore, fresh foods that have not been processed are the best for our overall health.

The processing of foods diminishes the healing power. Fresh fruits and vegetables give us an opportunity to reach peak wellbeing as well as assisting in the treatment of many common ailments that will present in daily life.

This text offers the reader an opportunity to use the powerful healing properties found in fruits and vegetables for both the prevention and treatment, of common ailments.

In clinical practice I see common conditions that could be assisted with specific fruit and vegetables being introduced as medicines, to the client's diet.

The cost factor is kept to a minimum with this type of treatment and the safety factor is unsurpassed in the realm of medicine. The healing ability and the powerful components found in these foods, is a wonderful study of natural medicines made available via nature.

Dr Sandi Rogers ED.D., N.D

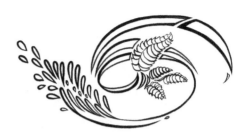

How To Use The Book

This book is intended to be an easy reference for the use of fruits and vegetables in the treatment of and assistance with, common ailments. It is not intended that you try all the treatments suggested for each ailment. Choose those best suited to you or your client. Availability of some fruits and vegetables may be seasonal, however, as many alternatives are offered using a fresh product will not be a problem.

The information contained in this text is presented as information only. It should not take the place of professional advice. Always consult your wholistically trained health care practitioner.

It is important to also note that depending on the condition being treated, it may be necessary to use the treatments recommended in conjunction with other medications, as prescribed by your medical practitioner, or wholistically trained natural therapist. Fruit and vegetables will offer many solutions to aid your wellbeing recovery.

The format of the book is very easy to follow and you may seek either as little or as much information as you need, or want, regarding which fruit and/or vegetable to use for a particular ailment and why it is the recommended treatment.

In this edition several products have been added, some not fruit and vegetables, however these products are useful. I can testify to their efficacy as they have been trialled in clinic by literally thousands of people, proving fruits and vegetables are truly a wonderful medicine.

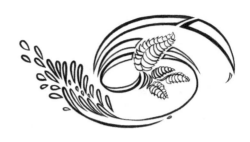

The Format Of The Book

SECTION ONE: COMMON AILMENTS

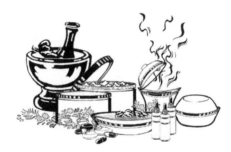

This section contains a series of common ailments, listed in alphabetical order for easy reference.

You simply look up the ailment you are wishing to treat and either one, or a number of suggested treatments, will be listed. Any recipes you may need will be referenced and easy to locate in Section Two.

SECTION TWO: FRUITS AND VEGETABLES

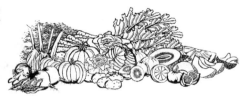

This section of the book contains a list of all the fruits and vegetables referred to in Section One. All fruits and vegetables are listed in alphabetical order for easy reference.

The information about each fruit and vegetable listed contains:

A. General information regarding each fruit and vegetable. It should be noted that this text focuses on the major constituents found within each fruit and vegetable and not every constituent is listed.

B. The key minerals, vitamins, acids and other nutrients each food contains.

C. Any recipes, specific cooking methods and instructions for any specific preparations, that might be suggested in Section One.

SECTION THREE: NUTRITIONAL ELEMENTS

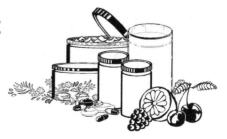

This section addresses all the nutritional elements referred to in Section Two, alphabetically listed, under the headings Minerals, Vitamins, Acids and Other Nutrients.

Information is provided regarding the action of each element and its healing effects on the body.

SECTION FOUR: HERBAL TEAS

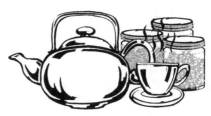

This section alphabetically lists all the herbal teas recommended in the treatment of various ailments in Section One. The information provides instructions as to where each tea can be purchased or alternatively, if you have to prepare it yourself, the recipe is provided.

SECTION FIVE: OIL TREATMENTS

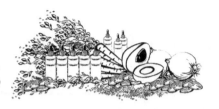

This section has alphabetically listed all the oil treatments referred to in Section One. A brief outline is given explaining the healing properties of each oil, which oil combinations are the most effective when treating specific conditions, and details of either where to purchase each oil, or how to prepare it yourself: whilst it is acknowledged that some oils are derived from plants other than fruit or vegetable, it was thought necessary to include them if the treatments suggested were to be as comprehensive as possible.

SECTION SIX: SMOOTHIES AND JUICES

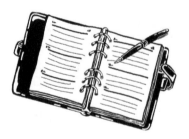

This section is a new addition to this update. Juices and smoothies have become very popular and quite trendy, yet most formulas offered are far too complex and phyto-chemically concentrated. It is essential that blends are balanced and in such concentrations not to overwhelm the body.

It is important to note that everything we consume has to be broken down and assimilated by the body. It is a delicate balance and 'less is more' should be considered when combining fruit, vegetables and grains.

Table of Contents

ACKNOWLEDGMENTS..**5**

DEDICATION..**6**

INTRODUCTION..**9**

HOW TO USE THE BOOK **11**

THE FORMAT OF THE BOOK **13**

    Section One: Common Ailments 13

    Section Two: Fruits and Vegetables 14

    Section Three: Nutritional Elements...................... 15

    Section Four: Herbal Teas 15

    Section Five: Oil Treatments................................... 16

    Section Six: Smoothies and Juices 16

SECTION ONE – COMMON AILMENTS **33**

  COMMON AILMENTS 34

    Introduction... 34

  ABSCESSES 36

    On the skin 36

    On the gums 37

  ACIDIC CONDITIONS 38

    General 38

    Excess uric acid... 39

  ANAEMIA... 42

    Anaemia in pregnancy.. 43

  ANXIETY.. 45

  APPETETE... 47

    To Increase/Stimulate 47

ARTERIOSCLEROSIS 48
ARTHRITIS 49
ASTHMA 51
    To assist in the prevention of asthma 52
BAD BREATH 53
BLADDER HEALTH 54
BLEEDING GUMS 55
BLOOD DISORDERS 56
    Coagulation 56
    The need for blood purifying 57
BLOOD PRESSURE 58
    HIGH 58
    LOW 59
BONES 60
    STRENGTHENING 60
BOILS 61
BOWEL HEALTH 62
    Regularity 62
    The cholesterol saga 63
    The elimination of gas pockets 66
BRONCHITIS 68
    General treatment 68
CANCER 70
    Help with the side affects of treatment 70
    As a defence against 70
CANDIDA 73
CARPAL TUNNEL 74
CATARRAH 75

CELIAC.. 76

CHOLESTEROL.. 78

   The breaking down of the arterial plaque that
   forms on the arterial wall 79

CHRONIC FATIGUE SYNDROME 80

COLD HANDS AND COLD FEET 82

CONJUNCTIVITIS.. 84

CONSTIPATION AND BOWEL DISORDERS
(COLITIS, DIVERTICULITIS) 85

CONVALESCENCE FROM A DISEASE............................ 87

CORTISONE TREATMENT.. 89

   The side effects (toxic build-up, fluid retention).... 89

   The effect on white blood cells 90

COUGHING.. 91

CRACKED HEELS 92

CYSTITIS... 93

DANDRUFF 94

DEPRESSION 95

DIABETES Type 11... 96

DIABETIC PERIPHERAL NEUROPATHY.......................... 98

DIARRHOEA 99

   Infantile.. 100

   Adult (with mucous or inflammation of
   the bowel)... 101

DIGESTION 102

   GAS 105

   The need to stabilise the function of the stomach 105

EAR ACHE 106

ECZEMA 107

EMOTIONAL INSTABILITY 108
IRRITABILITY 109
EMPHYSEMA 110
EYE TONER 111

FATIGUE/LOW LEVELS OF PHYSICAL AND
   MENTAL ENERGY 112
FLUID RETENTION 114
FOOD POISONING 115
GALL BLADDER DYSFUNCTION 116
GENERAL POOR HEALTH 117
GOUT 118
HAIR LOSS 121
HAIR SCALP (dry) 122
HAY FEVER 123
HEADACHE 125
HEARTBURN 126
HEART HEALTH 127
     Palpitations 128
     Tired heart syndrome 128
HEPATITIS 129
HERPES 130
HORMONAL RELATED CONDITIONS 131
     Sugar cravings 131
     Fluid retention 131
INDIGESTION 132
INFECTION 133
     Recurrent in children 133
     Intestinal 133

INFLAMMATION 134

INFLUENZA (COLDS, FLU) 136

COUGHING 138

INSECT BITES 139

    Reaction to insect bites 140

INSOMNIA 141

IRON – low 142

IRRITABILITY 143

IRRITABLE COLON 144

KIDNEY CONDITIONS 145

    Pain relief 145

    Promoting normal kidney function 145

    Stones 146

LACTATION 147

    To decrease 147

    To promote 147

LARYNGITIS 148

LIBIDO - LOW 149

LIVER DISORDERS 150

    Liver cell regeneration 150

    Liver and de-tox help 151

    Liver and increase bile flow 152

LUMBAGO 153

MOUTH ULCERS 154

MENSTRUATION 155

    Cramps 155

    Irregularity 155

MIGRAINES 156

MOTION SICKNESS 158

MUSCLE HEALTH 159

    Muscle aches.. 159

NAILS.. 160

    Ridging.. 160

    Splitting 160

NAPPY RASH.. 161

    Urine scalding.. 161

NAUSEA.. 162

NIGHT BLINDNESS... 163

PAIN CONTROL (AN ANALGESIC)................... 164

    Pain in the joints.. 164

PERIODS... 165

PREGNANCY 166

    Morning sickness.. 166

RESPIRATORY PROBLEMS............................... 167

    Excessive mucous 167

RESTLESS LEGS 168

RETARDED GROWTH 169

    Children 169

RHEUMATISM 170

RING WORM 171

SHINGLES 172

SINUS CONGESTION 173

SKIN CONDITIONS... 174

    Acne 174

    Acne due to poor diet 175

    Bad complexion... 175

Black heads.. 175

Burns.. 176

Burns - skin repair... 176

Chaffed/dry... 177

Damaged skin.. 177

Dry, scaly 178

Facial neuralgia (nerve pain of the face) 178

Facial steams - (cleanser) 179

Facial steams — (stimulator/toning).................... 179

Inflammation 179

Itching.. 179

Promoting elimination via the skin by
   increasing perspiration 180

SMELLY FEET 181

SPASM AND/OR INFLAMMATION OF THE STOMACH 182

STRESS 183

STYES... 184

SUGAR CRAVINGS... 185

THROAT CONDITIONS 186

Excess mucous 186

Inflammation and/or spasms of the throat and
   respiratory system....................................... 187

Sore throat 187

THRUSH 189

Thrush in the mouth 190

TINEA... 191

Mild cases 191

Stubborn cases 191

TIRED LEG SYNDROME 192

TISSUE FIRMING – 193

    Face, neck, breasts, abdomen and
      the wrinkling associated with post pregnancy.. 193

TONSILITIS 194

TOXAEMIA 195

    Toxin release from the body - assisting with 195

ULCERS IN THE DIGESTIVE SYSTEM 197

    Ulcers in the mouth 197

    Ulcers in the stomach 198

URINARY TRACT - Gravel In The Urine 199

    Urinary tract - infection 200

    Urinary tract -inflammation 201

    Urinary tract - maintaining a fluid balance 201

    Urinary tract - promoting the elimination of fluid 201

    Urinary tract - spasm 202

    Urinary tract - urinary sugar 202

VAGINAL THRUSH 203

VITAMIN C DEFICIENCY 204

WARTS 205

WORMS - INTESTINAL PARASITES 206

WOUNDS - PARTICULARLY THOSE DIFFICULT
    OR SLOW TO HEAL 207

SECTION TWO – FRUIT AND VEGETABLES 209

FRUIT AND VEGETABLES 210

ALFALFA SPROUTS - Medicago sativa 211

ALMONDS -Prunus amygdalus. 212

    Almond Milk Recipe 213

Almond Puree 214

APPLES–Malus communis 215

APRICOTS -Armenliaca vulgaris.............................. 217

    Reconstituting Dried Apricots 218

ASPARAGUS -Asparagus officinalis 219

AVOCADO –Persea gratissima 222

BANANA -Muser sapientum..................................... 225

BARLEY –Hordeum vulgare 228

BEANS -Phaseolus vulgaris 230

BEETROOT - Beta ruba 233

BLACKBERRIES –Rubus fructicosus...................... 235

    Blackberry Root Powder................................... 236

    Dried Blackberry Formula 237

BROCCOLI -Brassica oleracea italica 238

CABBAGE -Brassica oleracea 241

CALENDULA FLOWERS –Calendula officinalis 243

CANTALOUPE Cucumis melo................................ 244

CARROT–Daucus carota.. 245

CAULIFLOWER -Brassica oleracea 248

CAYENNE –Capsicum annum.................................. 250

    Cayenne Lotion... 251

CELERY –Apium graveolens 252

CHERRIES -Cerasus vulgaris 254

CHILLI – Capsicum annum...................................... 256

CLOVES -Sygizium aromaticum.............................. 258

CORN -Zea mays 260

CUCUMBER –Cucumis melo 262

CURRANTS – Ribes nigrum 264

DANDELION -Taraxacum officinalis 266

    Dandelion Drink Recipe 267

DATES -Phoenix dactylifera 268

EGGPLANT -Solanum melongena 269

FENNEL Foeniculum vulgare 271

FIGS —Ficus carica 273

GARLIC -Allium sativum & ONION-Allium cepa 275

    Onion and Garlic Soup Recipe 279

    Onion Syrup Formula 279

    Onion and Honey Syrup Recipe 280

GINGER Zingiber officinalis 281

GLOBE ARTICHOKE—Cynara scolymus 283

GRAPEFRUIT -Citrus decumana 285

HORSERADISH —Armoracia rusticana 287

KALE—Brassica oleracea var. sabellia 289

KIWI FRUIT—Actinidia chinensis 291

LEMON -Citrus limonum 293

    Lemon and Honey Syrup 294

    Roasted lemons 294

LETTUCE—Lactuca sativa 295

LOQUAT-Eriobotrya japonica 297

LYCEE Litchi clunenses 299

MANGO Mangifera indica 300

OLIVE—Olea europaea 301

ORANGE -Citrus auranrium 303

PARSLEY—Apium petroselinum 305

PAWPAW -Carica papaya 307

PEAR Pyrus commmunis 309

PEPPERMINT LEAVES—Mentha piperita 311

PINEAPPLE—Ananas sativus.. 312

POMEGRANATE—Punica granatum 314

POTATO -Solanum tuberosum.. 315

PRUNES—Prunus domestica.. 317

PUMPKIN SEEDS AND PUMPKIN —Cucurbita pepo 319

RADISH—Raphanus gativas 321

RHUBARB—Rhuem rhaponticum.................................. 323

ROLLED OATS —Avena sativa 325

    Oat Milk Recipe.. 326

SORRELL—Rumex 2acetosa 327

    Sorrel Bouillon Recipe 329

SPROUTS 330

STAWBERRIES—Fragaria ananassa 332

SWEET POTATO—Batatas batatas................................ 334

SPINACH—Spinacia oleracea 335

TOMATO—Solanum lycopersicum................................ 337

TURNIP -Brassica napus.. 339

WATERCRESS - Nasturtium officinale.......................... 340

WATERMELON—Cucurbita citrullus............................. 341

SECTION THREE – NUTRITIONAL ELEMENTS............... 343

VITAMINS, MINERALS AND OTHER NUTRIENTS......... 344

    Vitamins:.. 344

    Minerals: 357

    Acids: 366

    Other nutrients:... 368

SECTION FOUR – HERBAL TEAS AND SPICES 373

    Alfalfa tea 374

Aniseed tea 374

Apple cider and ginger beverage 374

Apple cider vinegar, ginger and
    peppermint beverage 375

Apple cider and lemon tea 375

Apple peel tea 375

Black currant tea 376

Blackberry tea 376

Blackberry leaf tea 376

Caraway seed tea 377

Chamomile tea 377

Coriander as a spice 377

Corn silk tea 377

Couch-grass tea 378

Dandelion root tea 378

Fennel tea 378

Fenugreek tea 378

Gin-soaked raisin remedy 378

Ginger tea 379

Ginger and lemon tea 380

Green bean pod tea 380

Hawthorn berry tea 381

Hops 381

Jasmine tea 381

Lemon balm tea 381

Oatmilk 382

Loquat leaf tea 382

Meadowsweet tea 382

Onion syrup... 383

Parsley tea 383

Peppermint tea 384

Raspberry leaf tea... 384

Sage tea.. 384

Slippery elm tea... 385

Thyme tea 385

Walnut tea 385

Watermelon seed tea.. 386

Yarrow tea 386

SECTION FIVE – OIL TREATMENTS............................. 387

OIL TREATMENTS.. 388

Avocado oil... 388

Cabbage ointment... 389

Carrot oil... 389

Coconut oil... 390

Lavender oil.. 390

Onion oil... 393

Sweet almond oil... 394

Tea tree oil.. 395

Thyme oil 396

SECTION SIX – JUICES AND SMOOTHIES.................... 397

Blends.. 402

Energiser 402

Internal cleanser.. 402

Immune booster... 402

Digestive aid 402

Immune activator... 403

Immune support 403

Skin cleanser 403

Blood tonic 403

Lung cleanser 1 404

Lung cleanser 2 404

Heart support (1) 404

Heart support (2) 405

Energy booster 405

Wellbeing recovery tonic 405

Liver tonic 405

Fluid remover 406

Muscle health (1) 406

Bowel health (1) 407

Bowel health (2) 407

Bowel health (3) 407

Immune support Viral invader 408

Immune support Viral destroyer 408

Immune health tonic (1) 408

Immune health tonic (2) 408

Memory booster 409

Arthritis pain reducer 409

Pain relief 410

Tummy soother (1) 410

Insomnia 411

Nervine tonic 411

Good health tonic 411

Liver health 411

Hay-fever help (1) 412

Hay-fever help (2) 412
Lower blood pressure... 412
Insomnia soother 412
Urinary tract cleanse 413
Eye health... 413
Fuel up tonic 413
Illness recovery... 414
Cold and flu recovery.. 414
Cholesterol lowering.. 415

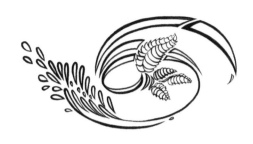

Section One
Common Ailments

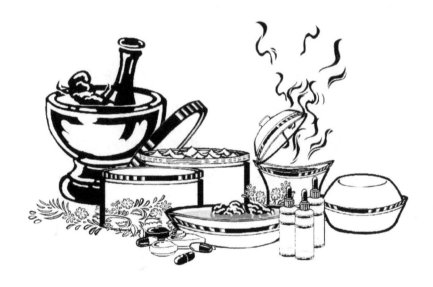

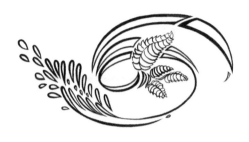

COMMON AILMENTS

Introduction

With all conditions it is essential you consider if you have any food sensitivities. Many conditions flare up as foods enter the body and as there is a sensitivity to the food the body struggles. This does not mean to say the food is a 'bad' food rather you simply have a sensitivity. I have many clients who are sensitive to apples and as we all know *'an apple a day keeps the doctor away'* or does it? So how would one know if there is a sensitivity?

Ask yourself how you feel when you consume foods. Do you feel bloated or slightly nauseous? Your body may be struggling. This can happen with even the very best food.

Keep a food diary and your physical response linked to a time line. This can be of great benefit in particular if you consult with a natural medicine consultant who follows the tradition of natural medicine and has not fallen into the trap of using lots of pills and potions. They will be able to guide you into the wonderful world of fruit and vegetables as medicine.

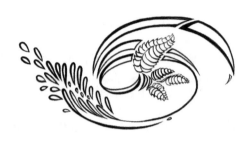

ABSCESSES

On the skin

1 – Place grated, raw potato over the abscess and cover with gauze - tape plastic wrap over gauze and let draw. Tape to seal.

2 – Dip a cabbage leaf into boiling water and apply to the abscess. Cover with gauze or lightly bandage and let draw.

3 – The preparation of a poultice, made by the splitting and soaking of a dry fig in warm water for a few minutes and then applying it to the abscess, will reduce inflammation. Cover and allow to draw.

4 – Moisten powdered tapioca, apply it to the abscess, cover and allow it to draw. (Powdered tapioca can be purchased at supermarkets or delicatessens).

5 - Pulp raw onion or garlic and place on the abscess, cover with gauze or a light bandage and let draw. You can also cover with plastic wrap to create a seal; if it becomes too painful take the plastic wrap off, allow the pain to settle and start again when comfortable to do so.

6 - Powder carrot seeds to make a teaspoon, add apple cider vinegar to form a paste and apply to the area. Cover with gauze.

On the gums

1 - Abscesses on the gums may respond to the placing of a fresh or dried fig over the area in the mouth.

2 - Make carrot seeds into a paste and massage into the gums using the above combination.

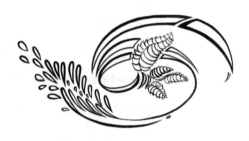

ACIDIC CONDITIONS

General

1 – Introduce cherries regularly into your diet. When in season place the whole cherries into freezer trays and cover with water. Freeze and defrost as needed.

2 – Introduce figs regularly into your diet.

3 – Introduce celery regularly into your diet.

4 – Introduce potato juice. Simply peel one potato and juice. Drink juice to settle

5 – Introduce papaya or pawpaw into the diet.

6 – Drink meadowsweet tea (See Section Four).

7 – A good combination of foods to introduce are:

– guavas

– bell peppers

– papaya

- baby corn
- red cabbage
- onions
- apples
- oranges
- strawberries
- olives

8 - Although not a fruit nor vegetable start to include bi-carbonate of soda daily. Use only a pinch a day and ensure it is aluminium free.

9 - Apple cider vinegar, ginger and peppermint is an effective combination. To 500mls of Apple Cider Vinegar add 2 tablespoons of fresh grated ginger and 1 cup of crushed peppermint leaves (or common mint). Allow to stand for 1 day. Take 10mls of the blended vinegar with 50mls of water. Allow ginger and mint to be in the liquid as you drink. No need to strain.

Excess uric acid

1 - Introduce the juice of half a cucumber, in combination with the juice of half a carrot, into your daily diet. Begin with 50% of each

but if you need more fluid elimination then increase the cucumber. If there is any infection or inflammation, in the body, then you would increase the carrot juice.

2 – To assist in alkalising, drink 500mls. of barley water daily. (Barley water can be purchased from the supermarket or alternatively soak barley overnight in water and strain).

3 – Introduce two grated apples, including the peel, into your daily diet. Continue this treatment until condition clears.

4 – Infuse one teaspoon of either grated apple or grapefruit peel in boiling water and sip to settle acid stomach.

5 – Eat half an avocado when suffering from an acidic gut or heart burn.

6 – Drink a wine glass of potato juice.

7 – Drink celery juice, or alternatively, eat four cubes of pawpaw or one slice of pineapple.

8 – Drink apple peel tea (See Section Four).

*All the above recommendations may be used regularly.

Dietary considerations are:

> increase fluid intake.

> eliminate alcohol.

> reduce fat intake.

> reduce protein intake.

> reduce purines in diet.

Common purine foods are organ meats, meats, shell fish, yeast, herrings, mackerel.

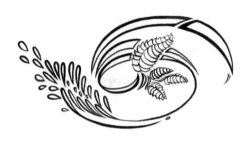

ANAEMIA

1 – Introduce apricots into your diet. As they have a short season use dried apricots and hydrate by placing them in a glass of water, leave overnight, drink the water and eat the fruit.

2 – Introduce asparagus into your diet.

3 – Modern herbalists use the blackberry root, due to the iron content, to help treat this condition. Use one teaspoon of powdered blackberry root to a cup of hot water and drink daily. (Refer to Blackberries in Section Two for the method used to powder the blackberry root).

4 – Introduce cabbage regularly into your diet.

5 – Introduce celery regularly into your diet.

6 – Introduce corn regularly into your diet.

7 – Introduce eggplant regularly into your diet

8 - Include Vitamin C enriched foods with meals. (Refer to Section Two to help identify these foods).

9 - Introduce lettuce into the diet

10 - Introduce pumpkin into the diet

◑ NOTE

---

*note meat, fish and poultry are the best source of haem iron

*It is important to note that you should not drink tea or coffee with any meals, particularly if suffering from anaemia - wait at least an hour.

Anaemia in pregnancy

Normally the iron requirement during pregnancy is approximately 27mgs.

1 - Introduce avocado into your diet. This will also help the unborn child to develop healthy skin, bones and teeth.

2 – Alfalfa sprouts are very nutritious and a good source of iron for the mother to be.

3 – Eat all berries as they are high in iron.

4 – Eat Vitamin C rich foods at the same time as eating iron rich foods.

5 – Introduce foods as indicated under anaemia.

6 – See blood tonic

7 – Include products listed in upper section.

◑ **NOTE**

---

*note meat, fish and poultry are the best source of haem iron

*It is important to note that you should not drink tea or coffee with any meals, particularly if suffering from anaemia - wait at least an hour.

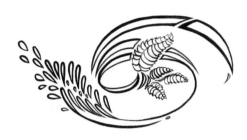

ANXIETY

1 – Introduce apples into your diet, either juiced, grated, pulped or whole, making sure that the peel is also included.

2 – Introduce half an avocado into your diet every second day. This is particularly effective if mixed with apple.

3 – Introduce broccoli into your diet.

4 – Introduce beetroot into the diet

5 – Introduce corn into your diet.

6 – Introduce eggplant into your diet.

7 – Eat rolled oats for breakfast.

8 – Drink oat milk daily made by mixing 1 cup of uncooked rolled oats to 1 litre of water and leave in the fridge to infuse for about an hour. Shake

the contents and strain. Drink the milk over the course of the day leaving in fridge.

9 – Ensure that you are consuming adequate protein. Start the day with protein and have low fat proteins with each and every meal.

10 – Eat lettuce regularly.

◑ **Note**

It is essential you consider life circumstances and learn coping strategies linked with nutrition and work with a good mentor you feel comfortable with.

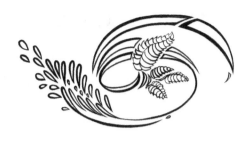

APPETETE

To Increase/Stimulate

1 – Eat apricots, preferably fresh, before a meal.

2 – Introduce globe artichoke into your diet, as a bitter tonic.

3 – Introduce juiced or steamed (not pickled) beetroot into your diet.

4 – When taken by itself celery acts as an appetite stimulant.

5 – Introduce bitter salad combination (purchased from most supermarkets and fruit shops) into your daily diet, preferably thirty minutes before meal time. Sprinkle with a small amount of lemon juice and or apple cider vinegar.

6 – Introduce avocado into the diet

ARTERIOSCLEROSIS

1 – Eat garlic regularly.

2 – Drink apple juice daily, making sure that the peel has also been juiced with the apple, or alternatively eat three apples a day.

3 – Introduce beetroot regularly into your diet.

4 – Eat half an avocado every second day.

5 – Introduce garlic and onion regularly into your diet, as they are renowned for assisting the heart and the arteries to remain healthy.

6 – Eat artichoke regularly.

7 – Eat ginger regularly.

8 – Drink hawthorn berry tea (See Section Four).

9 – Drink black tea, but not with meals.

10 – Make an apple cider vinegar and ginger beverage. See recipe Section four.

11 – Introduce chilli into the diet

12 – Introduce capsicum into the diet.

ARTHRITIS

1 - Drink 150mls.of apple juice daily, making sure that the peel has also been juiced with the apple.

2 - Alternate the apple juice with two cups of apple peel tea. (See to Section Four).

3 - Introduce asparagus into your diet three times a week.

4 - Introduce one banana into your daily diet.

5 - Drink a combination of the juice of one carrot, one apple and three sticks of celery. This should be taken twice daily.

6 - Eat ten blackberries daily. When in season place whole fruit in freezer trays, cover with water and freeze - defrost as needed.

7 - Eat cherries regularly - freeze as in blackberry and defrost as needed.

8 - Drink apple cider vinegar and lemon tea (Refer to Tea Section—Four).

9 - Avoid sugar and reduce, (not cut out) inflammatory foods. These are:

- Red meat

- Potato

- High dairy intake

Remove

- Diet soft drinks
- Sugar supplements
- White flour products

Include anti-inflammatory foods. These are:

- Cherries
- Apples
- Blueberries and most berries
- Sweet potato
- Leafy greens such as kale (always steam first) and spinach
- Artichokes
- Green, red, pinto beans
- Carrot
- Figs
- Celery
- Barley

◑ **Note**

See Section Four for Gin – Soaked Raisin Remedy

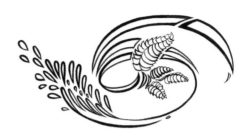

ASTHMA

1 - Drink almond milk. This is recommended as a. treatment, if you are prone to this condition, then drink it daily as a preventive measure. (Refer to Almond in Section Two for Almond Milk recipe). *It is important to note that this is meant as a complementary formula and should be taken in conjunction with those medicines prescribed by your medical practitioner.*

2 - Place a cabbage poultice onto your chest

3 - Drink 1 part cabbage and 2 parts carrot juice daily.

4 - Drink warmed carrot juice.

5 - Wrap a peeled garlic clove in a small amount of bread and swallow whole, daily.

6 - Eat 3 constituted dried apricots a day. Soak

overnight in water and consume the apricots and water the following morning.

7 - Onion syrup may assist (See Section Four).

8 - A formulation that works well as a complementary medicine for asthma is a combination of 50% carrot juice, 25% apple juice and 25% onion juice.

To assist in the prevention of asthma

1 - Eat horseradish. This can be eaten as a complementary addition to a main meal.

2 - Introduce figs into your diet.

3 - Take onion syrup daily. Dosage: children 1 teaspoon, adults 1 tablespoon. (Refer to Garlic and Onion in Section Two for Onion Syrup recipe).

4 - Introduce sorrel into your diet.

5 - Eat onion and garlic to keep chest clear.

6 - Eat leafy green vegetables.

7 - Drink any of the immune juice or smoothie combinations (See Section Six).

BAD BREATH

◑ Caution

The following treatments are suggested assuming that all the conventional avenues, investigation of the mouth, teeth and the gastro-intestinal tract, have been exhausted and the condition remains.

---

1 – Eat bitter salad combination (purchased from most supermarkets and fruit shops).

2 – Eating a few cubes of pawpaw prior to a meal will assist the digestive process by enhancing assimilation and elimination.

3 – Introduce two apples into your daily diet, remembering to include the skin.

4 – Drink chamomile tea or peppermint tea on a regular basis (See Section Four).

5 – Drink one tablespoon of apple cider vinegar (purchased from a health food store).

6 – Drink digestion smoothies and juice daily (See Section Six).

BLADDER HEALTH

Once the bladder weakens it is essential to support the entire urinary tract by entering into the diet foods that can offer healing. One point that has to be emphasised is the therapeutic use of water; sip across the day to avoid dehydration and aid the flushing mechanism to work.

1 - Introduce watercress.
2 - Introduce cranberries.
3 - Introduce leeks.
4 - Introduce olives.
5 - Introduce cherries.
6 - Introduce apples.
7 - Introduce carrots.
8 - Introduce parsley.
9 - Introduce celery

Mix and match these products to aid the function of the bladder (See Section Six for a urinary blend).

BLEEDING GUMS

◑ **Caution**

It is important to note that these recommenda-tions should be taken in conjunction with those medicines prescribed by your medical practitioner or your qualified natural medicine consultant.

---

1 – The eating of raw cauliflower has been reputed to assist with this condition.

2 – Rinse the mouth with cucumber and carrot juice.

3 – Blackberries may assist to stop bleeding and tone up gums.

4 – Rinse mouth with carrot juice as an anti-infective.

5 – Apply a small amount of cayenne pepper directly onto bleeding gum. This will sting, but it will stop the bleeding.

6 – Rinse mouth with pure lemon juice.

7 – Drink the juice of a carrot include the top rinsing around the mouth then swallowing.

8 – Drink pomegranate juice daily.

BLOOD DISORDERS

1 - Eat all berries as a general tonic for the blood, as they are high in iron.

2 - Introduce kiwi fruit into your diet as it is good for the circulatory system.

Coagulation

1 - Introduce asparagus into your diet.

2 - Drink 250mls of cabbage juice daily.

3 - Introduce either dried or fresh apricots into your daily diet.

4 - Introduce a cup of green beans into your daily diet — juiced or steamed.

5 - The regular introduction of raw celery into your diet helps to build healthy blood cells.

6 - Parsley acts as an excellent blood purifier and builder and should be introduced regularly into your diet.

7 - Introduce fresh garlic regularly into your diet.

8 - Introduce two apples into your daily diet, either juiced or whole, making sure that the peel is also included.

9 - Introduce raw cauliflower into your diet.

10 – Drink pomegranate juice regularly.

The need for blood purifying

1 – Introduce raw onions into your diet at least three times a week.

2 – Introduce garlic regularly into your diet.

3 – Introduce grapefruit juice into your daily diet. Remember to always include the skin as it is high in the essential oils that help cleanse the body.

4 – Parsley acts as an excellent blood purifier and builder and should be introduced regularly into your diet.

5 – Drink apple cider vinegar and lemon tea. Simply add 1 teaspoon of Apple Cider Vinegar and the juice of a ¼ lemon to a cup of boiling water.

6 – Drink pomegranate juice regularly.

◑ **Note**

For information on diabetes refer to diabetes in: section one

---

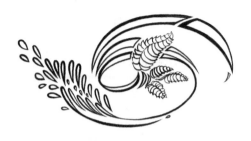

BLOOD PRESSURE

1 – Introduce three apples into your daily diet, either juiced or whole, making sure that the peel is also included.

2 – Cucumber, because of its potassium levels, is suitable for the treatment of both high and low blood pressure.

3 – Introduce coriander into the diet in powder form (derived from the seeds) and or the leaves in cooking and salads.

4 – Introduce pomegranate juice and whole fruit into the diet.

HIGH

1 – Introduce onion into your diet.

2 – Introduce a cup of beans into your daily diet to help lower blood pressure. This is particularly effective

where there is fluid retention associated with B.P.

3 – Introduce broccoli regularly into your diet.

4 – Introduce carrot regularly into your diet.

5 – Eat one clove of garlic daily. To avoid the odour take a whole clove of garlic, peel it and wrap it in a piece of bread. Take as a tablet.

6 – Consume kiwi fruit regularly due to potassium and balanced sodium content.

7 – Introduce a small amount of spicy food into your diet.

8 – Introduce raw beetroot into the diet in small amounts on a daily basis. Grated, tossed through salads are quite palatable.

9 – Introduce pomegranate juice into the diet.

LOW

1 – Introduce three figs into your diet. You may soak dried figs in water overnight to reconstitute them before eating.

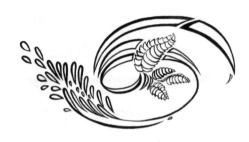

BONES

STRENGTHENING

1 – Introduce one fully ripened banana into your daily diet.

2 – Maintain a diet high in fresh unprocessed foods and restrict salty, sugary and fatty foods.

3 – Exercise and add weights such as wearing a back pack with a few bricks included (weight to be comfortable, start low and slow).

BOILS

1. Apply a cabbage poultice to the affected area.
2. The preparation of a poultice, made by the splitting open and soaking of a dried fig in warm water for a few minutes and then applying it to the boil, will reduce inflammation.
3. Apply grated, raw potato over the boil. Cover with gauze or light bandage and allow to draw.
4. Place bread over the boil and allow to draw.
5. Place raw onion over the boil. Cover with gauze or a light bandage and allow to draw.
6. Mash together one clove of crushed garlic and half a teaspoon of oil. Place over the boil and cover with gauze, or a light bandage, and allow to draw.
7. Drink any immune juice or smoothie (See Section Six).
8. Make a poultice using carrot seeds that have been soaked in a small amount of apple cider vinegar and made into a paste. Apply to the boil.

▶ Ensure a good balance with nutrition by eating fresh fruits and vegetables daily.

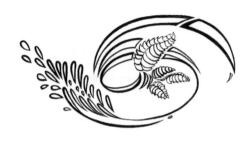

BOWEL HEALTH

(also see coeliac)

Regularity

1 – Eat fifteen almonds daily (preferably roasted).

2 – Drink eight to ten glasses of water daily. Drink in small amounts over the whole day and add a few slices of lemon.

3 – Eat one apple, including the peel, first thing every morning. Grate apple if preferred.

4 – Introduce three grated apples into your daily diet, making sure that the peel is also included.

5 – The introduction of one cup of green beans into your daily diet, will aid in normal bowel function, due to their fibrous content.

6 – Introduce cabbage regularly into your diet.

7 – Soak three prunes overnight in half a glass of

water and the juice of one lemon. In the morning eat the prunes and drink the juice.

8 –   The drinking of a bouillon made using sorrel can work as a laxative. (Refer to Sorrel in Section Two for the bouillon recipe. Please read the cautions listed as there are some conditions in which sorrel can be harmful).

9 –   Eat 2 kiwi fruit <u>including the peel</u> each day.

10 –   Eat loquats when in season.

11 –   Eat mangoes when in season.

12 –   Drink apple cider vinegar and lemon juice daily. Start with 5mls of apple cider vinegar and juice of ¼ lemon and 50mls of water,.

The cholesterol saga

There is so much confusion in the marketplace as people struggle to lower their cholesterol. The first thing is to understand the terms that are used and what they mean without creating any further confusion. The three components you must be aware of are:

> LDL (the bad guy)

> HDL (the good guy)

> Triglycerides (bad guy)

When given a total reading it is imperative you know the levels of LDL and Triglycerides. Ask your practitioner to explain these elements to you and if they require a reduction then food, fabulous food can come to the rescue; or be a major cause of why your body is having trouble. By reducing bad fats, reducing or eliminating cow's milk and products and eliminating as much sugar as you can you will be well on your way to controlling cholesterol. In addition you must make sure your bowel is regularly evacuated as constipation can be a major problem if you have elevated cholesterol.

1 - Introduce garlic and onion into your diet.

2 - Introduce three grated apples into your daily diet, making sure that the peel is also included.

3 - Introduce globe artichoke into your diet three times a week. Introduce asparagus into your diet.

4 - Introduce dandelion leaves into your diet by

eating them in a salad.

5 – Introduce pear juice into your daily diet.

6 – Reduce fats and sugars from the diet and increase the variety of fresh fruit and vegetables. Up to 30 varieties of foods and the more colourful the better. What! I can hear you yelling as you peer over the rim of you glasses. Yes 30. Think about it. Let us take a salad. You may use:

- Lettuce
- Tomato
- Cucumber
- Celery
- Beetroot
- Olives
- Mushroom
- Grated apple
- Slice of orange
- Walnuts
- Egg
- Chicken or fish
- Olive oil, lemon and balsamic dressing
- There is 50% of the 30 varieties. easy!

7 - Enter barley in the form of pearl barley, barley grass, barley green powder.

8 - Introduce avocado into the diet.

9 - Introduce rolled oats into the diet.

10 - Introduce raw beetroot into the diet.

11 - Introduce chilli into the diet.

12 - Introduce cholesterol lowering smoothies and juices (See Section Six).

13 - Introduce pomegranate fruit and juice into the diet.

The elimination of gas pockets

1 - Introduce beetroot into your diet.

2 - The relief from excessive gas, caused through slow digestion, can be gained by drinking equal parts of carrot and apple juice.

3 - Drink the juice of one potato. This can be combined with carrot juice if you wish.

4 - Eat parsley.

5 - The drinking of the following teas assists in the elimination of gas: peppermint, chamomile and fennel (See Section Four).

6 - Apple cider vinegar and fresh ginger grated offers a powerhouse of healing. Take 1 teaspoon of apple cider vinegar, add 1 tablespoon of ginger to 50mls of water. Drink and eat ginger to add this combination to any of the digestive smoothies or juices recommended in section six.

7 - Chamomile, meadowsweet and or mint tea

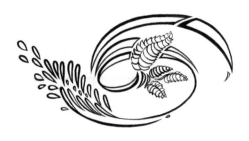

BRONCHITIS

General treatment

1 – Drink almond milk. (Refer to Almond in Section Two).

2 – Introduce garlic into your diet.

3 – Drink a combination of 40% each of carrot and apple juice and 20% asparagus juice, for chronic bronchitis. This should be warmed before drinking to avoid spasms that can result in drinking cold drinks when suffering from respiratory problems.

4 – Apply a cabbage poultice, onto the chest.

5 – Foods in combination eaten on a regular basis may assist, these are:

– horseradish

– capsicum

- pineapple
- orange
- honey
- dates
- cabbage
- onions
- figs

6 - Combination 50% carrot juice, 25% apple juice and 25% onion juice.

7 - Drink onion and garlic soup. (Refer to Garlic and Onion in Section Two).

8 - Slice and place onion onto bottom of feet, wrapping with bandages. Leave on the feet for several hours to relieve the condition.

9 - Honey and lemon juice (from the whole lemon including peel) when combined clears mucous. Combine 2/3 lemon and 1/3 honey in a small amount of warm water and consume three times daily.

10 - Drink apple juice, making sure that the peel has been juiced with the apple.

11 - Drink any immune juice or smoothie listed in section six under immune or respiration.

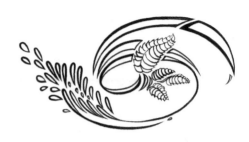

CANCER

Help with the side affects of treatment

1 – Introduce apples into the diet, making sure that the peel is also included, to help assist in the cleansing of the blood.

2 – Drink 200mls.of a combination of 50% carrot and 50% apple juice, daily.

3 – Eat globe artichoke to help cleanse the liver.

4 – Mash cooked sweet potato, pumpkin and avocado together as often the taste buds are affected and food tolerance is low.

As a defence against

Fruits and vegetables offer anti-carcinogenic support

1 – Introduce two apricots, either fresh or reconstituted dried apricots, into your daily diet.

These could also be linked in with carrot and celery juice. (Refer to Apricots in Section Two for the method used to reconstitute dried apricots).

2 - There is currently a study being done on the effective use of beans in the prevention of certain cancers. (Alexander Ferenczi M.D., Department of Internal Disease, Gsorna, Hungary, from Heinerman (p. 29).

3 - Beetroot has been found to work effectively as an anti-cancer agent.

4 - Pureed blackberry fruit has also been found to work effectively as an anti-cancer agent.

5 - Lots of fresh fruits and vegetables included in the diet and the elimination of highly processed foods.

6 - Good hydration is a must. Sip water regularly throughout the day, every day.

7 - Research in both 1983 and an extended study in 1989, showed that a half a cup of broccoli a day helped in the prevention of several cancers, particularly colonic and lung cancer. Prostate and Stomach Cancer also responded well to tests. It was also found that patients who had

Bowel Cancer and had undergone surgery, responded to the introduction of broccoli, cabbage and brussel sprouts when one or a combination of the three, was consumed three times per week. (US. National Cancer Institute Report (1987).

8 – International research has shown that broccoli can help in the prevention of Cervical Cancer. This research was first published in 1952 and has regularly been referred to in both science and medical journals.

9 – The regular intake of raw tomato has been scientifically validated as a cancer preventive. Research is continuing. See tomato.

10 – Drink immune smoothie or juices and mix and match the various products.

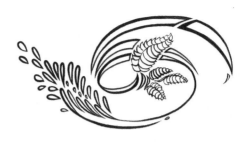

CANDIDA

Candida can be quite troublesome and many changes may need to be made to the diet, however these tips may assist the healing process.

1 – Introduce kohlrabi
2 – Introduce lettuce
3 – Eat natural yoghurt
4 – Introduce asparagus
5 – Introduce cabbage
6 – Introduce kale (lightly steamed)
7 – Introduce avocado

◑ **Note**

It is important to take out starchy foods and sugar.

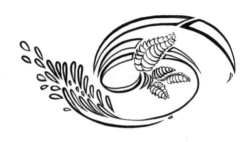

CARPAL TUNNEL

This condition can be quite debilitating and can get to the point a surgeon has to release the tendons. A few tips may assist in gaining some relief from the pain.

1 – Use a cabbage poultice. Freeze the outer leaves of the cabbage and each night wrap the wrist in the cabbage leaf, cover with gladwrap, place a bandage over the poultice and leave overnight.

2 – Drink parsley juice to reduce fluid build up.

3 – Drink celery juice to reduce fluid build up.

4 – Drink fresh pineapple juice to reduce fluid build up.

CATARRAH

1 – Introduce figs into your diet.

2 – Eat onion and garlic regularly.

3 – Drink onion and garlic soup. (Refer to Garlic and Onion in Section Two.)

4 – Eat horseradish. This can be eaten as a complementary addition to a main meal.

5 – Drink a combination of the juice of five cabbage leaves and the juice of one carrot. This is to be taken twice daily.

6 – Drink a combination of honey and lemon juice. Refer to bronchitis.

7 – Drink onion syrup - 1 tablespoon, 3 times a day. (Refer to Garlic and Onion in Section Two).

8 – Apple cider vinegar can assist with the reduction of mucous ensuring you take the vinegar that has the '*Mother*' in it. There will be a cloudy appearance.

9 – Eat turnips (lightly steamed).

10 – Drink lung tonic juice (See Section Six).

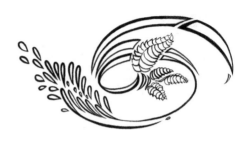

CELIAC

Clinical presentations of celiac disease is increasing. There appears to be a link between modern lifestyle where highly processed fast food, fast lifestyle and gluten rich foods are more evident.

Treatment must incorporate the entire lifestyle of the person in keeping with the tradition of natural medicine.

Celiac disease may be triggered by a sudden onset of stress, an intestinal infection or infestation of intestinal parasites, use of laxatives, sudden change in diet and or low levels of B 6.

Most celiac sufferers are malnourished due to the condition as absorption of nutrients is greatly restricted.

The following information may assist to get the assimilation and elimination improving and bring on comfort.

1 – Eat a gluten free diet that offers small amounts of highly nutritious fresh foods in order to get a full range of minerals, vitamins and nutrients.

2 – Exclude all cereals except for rice and corn to start with.

3 – Remove processed sugar from diet completely.

4 – Eat low fat proteins.

5 – Grate apple and carrot and eat daily.

6 – Introduce fruits and vegetables high in Vitamin B's (fortunately most offer B vitamins (check all fruit and vegetables in this book to see a wide range).

7 – See smoothie and juices for additional support. (See Section Six).

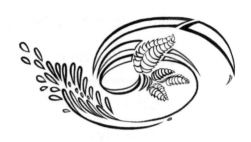

CHOLESTEROL

1 – Introduce three apples into your daily diet, either juiced or whole, making sure that the peel is also included.

2 – Take globe artichoke in a liquid formulation, as prescribed by a herbalist.

3 – Introduce four asparagus stalks into your daily diet.

4 – Medical scientists have been prescribing one cup of green beans per day, as part of their prescriptions, to help lower bad cholesterol. Statistically it has been found to lower LDL and triglycerides by at least 19% using beans as the only prescription. (Jean Carper, The Food Pharmacy, pg. 134- 135.)

5 – Introduce both garlic and onion regularly into your diet.

6 - Eat fresh oranges.

7 - Eat dandelion leaves as part of a salad, or drink dandelion root as a beverage. (Refer to Dandelion in Section Two for recipe).

8 - Drink black tea daily - no milk or sugar added.

9 - Drink jasmine tea.

10 - Introduce Barley into diet (see barley for variety).

11 - Introduce oats into the diet, blend with barley.

12 - Remove sugar and fats from the diet, being cautious about replacing full fat foods with low fat as the sugar content may be increased to compensate for the reduction of fat. Taste has to come from somewhere.

13 - Add spices and chilli to the diet to cleanse the blood.

The breaking down of the arterial plaque that forms on the arterial wall

1 - Take globe artichoke in a liquid formulation, as prescribed by a herbalist.

2 - Introduce turnips into your diet.

3 - Introduce both garlic and onions into your daily diet.

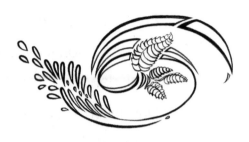

CHRONIC FATIGUE SYNDROME

◑ **Caution**

---

*It is important to note that this condition must first be professionally diagnosed by an wholistically trained health care professional, as many points must be confirmed before a correct diagnosis can be given.

---

1 –   Introduce three apples into your daily diet, either juiced or whole, making sure that the peel is also included.

2 –   Eat ten almonds daily (preferably roasted).

3 –   Introduce asparagus regularly into your diet.

4 –   Scientific testing in the United States has shown that this syndrome has been treated, with some

success, using the combination of banana and honey taken on a daily basis.

5 - Introduce bitter salad combination (purchased from most supermarkets and fruit shops) into you daily diet.

6 - Eat half an avocado daily.

7 - Introduce leafy green vegetables into your daily diet.

8 - Eat one banana daily.

9 - Ensure protein intake is adequate - include protein at each meal.

10 - Protein rich vegetable sources are mushrooms, beans and lentils to name a few.

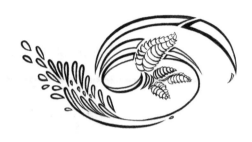

COLD HANDS AND COLD FEET

Warming foods are essential.

1 - These include ginger, radish and cayenne.
2 - The addition of potassium rich foods are also helpful. These include:

- Banana
- Coriander
- Apples
- Avocado
- Dates
- Figs
- Cabbage
- Baked beans
- Carrots
- Mushrooms
- Pumpkin

- Potato
- Tomatoes
- Lettuce
- Nuts and seeds

◑ **Note**

This is a small selection however there is enough of a selection to get you started.

Have your iron levels checked.

CONJUNCTIVITIS

1 - A regular intake of carrot juice for a short period of time will help break the cyclical pattern of this condition.

2 - Apply a cucumber slice to the eye after having dipped it in honey. Leave this on the eye for a few hours.

3 - Apply young cabbage leaves to the eye having dipped them in boiling water, and allowing them to cool. Leave on the eye for a few hours.

4 - Place dandelion leaves on the eye and leave for a few hours.

5 - Gently apply carrot oil on the condition. This oil is a very powerful healer and will aid rapid healing (See Section Five).

6 - Eat more fresh foods and less processed foods.

7 - Introduce immune smoothies or juices (See Section Six).

*Assess why conjunctivitis is occurring. Stress, compromised immune system and dehydration may have an affect.

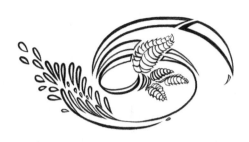

CONSTIPATION AND BOWEL DISORDERS (COLITIS, DIVERTICULITIS)

1 – Drink almond milk. (Refer to Almond in Section Two).

2 – Eat one grated apple, including peel, before bed. Also eat one grated apple, including peel, first thing in the morning, followed by the juice of half a lemon and a small amount of water.

3 – Eat five prunes left to sit overnight in 100mls. of water - eat the prunes and drink the liquid.

4 – Introduce asparagus into your diet.

5 – Introduce beans into your diet.

6 – Take on empty stomach. One teaspoon of powdered blackberry root, combined with a small amount of water. (Refer to Blackberries in

Section Two for the method used to powder the blackberry root).

7 – Introduce kiwi fruit into the diet ensuring you eat the peel as well. Blend is the best option.

8 – Introduce cabbage regularly into your diet if you have a tendency to suffer from constipation, or for the treatment of a bowel disease.

9 – Due to its natural fibre, grated carrot will aid in the treatment of constipation.

10 – Introduce cauliflower into your diet.

11 – Introduce figs into your diet. These are particularly effective if you drink the juice of the dried figs that have been soaked overnight.

12 – Drink pear juice regularly.

13 – Introduce pearl barley into the diet can mix with oats.

14 – Eat a mango a day. Due to short season these may be frozen by removing the skin cutting the cheeks off and freeze.

15 – Eat raw grated beetroot and mix with grated apple.

16 – Add cloves to food, juices or smoothies in small but regular amounts.

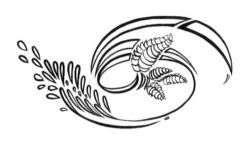

CONVALESCENCE FROM A DISEASE

1 – Drink almond milk once daily. (Refer to Almond in Section Two).

2 – Drink apple juice, making sure that the peel has been juiced with the apple.

3 – Eat three apricots daily, preferably fresh.

4 – Introduce five asparagus stalks into your daily diet.

5 – Introduce a cup of beans into your daily diet.

6 – Introduce cherries regularly into your diet.

7 – The high vitamin content of pineapple juice gives it the ability to support the immune system.

8 – Introduce parsley into your diet to help the immune system.

9 - Introduce grapefruit into your diet, to aid the immune system.

10 - Introduce sorrel into your diet. (Please read Sorrel in Section Two before eating it as there are some conditions in which sorrel can be harmful).

11 - Introduce raw vegetable juice daily (choose 3 different vegetables).

12 - See immune smoothies and juices (See Section Six).

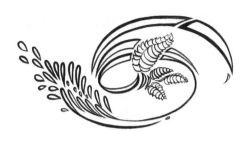

CORTISONE TREATMENT

The side effects (toxic build-up, fluid retention)

Cortisone is a vital treatment for many conditions. The side effects may be addressed using a sensible approach to linking conventional and natural medicines.

1 – Introduce three apples into your daily diet, either juiced or whole, making sure that the peel is also included.
2 – Introduce a cup of beans into your daily diet. Introduce dandelion leaf salad into your daily diet.
3 – Introduce grated, raw beetroot into your diet to assist liver cleansing.
4 – Introduce liver support juice and smoothies (See Section Six).

The effect on white blood cells

1 - Bean juice can help to counteract this side effect. You may combine beans with other vegetables, when juicing, such as carrot, apple and celery. The apple is of benefit to include because, apart from its nutritional value, it neutralises most of the flavours you may not like.

2 - Introduce raw fruit and vegetable juice daily.

3 - Choose immune smoothies or juices
(See Section Six)

COUGHING

1 – Eat blackberries, either whole or pulped, to soothe the throat.

2 – Eating a cup of whole, green beans, lightly steamed with a couple of cloves of garlic, to help address a troublesome, irritating cough.

3 – For a dry cough drink two parts cabbage juice and one part honey.

4 – Gargle and swallow 50mls. of cabbage juice, blended with honey to taste.

5 – Warmed carrot juice will help to breakdown the congestion that can form on the respiratory centre.

6 – Soak two dried figs overnight. In the morning eat the figs and drink the juice.

7 – Eat horseradish. This can be eaten as a complementary addition to a main meal.

8 – Sip onion juice and honey, using two parts onion juice and one part honey.

9 – Blend 1 part lemon juice, including peel, to 5 parts water and 1 part honey. Sip as needed.

10 – Drink lemon and honey syrup as needed. (Refer to Lemon in Section Two).

11 – Introduce 3 radishes and 1 apple juiced daily.

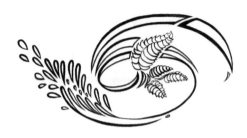

CRACKED HEELS

1 – Massage into feet the juice of 1 whole lemon, including peel, blended with 10mls of Vegetable based sorbalene massaged into heels.

2 – Make a paste with 1 whole lemon (include peel) with raw sugar. Massage into heels to soften dried or cracked skin.

◑ **Note**

If wearing open backed shoes it is absolutely imperative you moisturise the heels morning and night to maintain moist skin and help to reduce the trauma the flapping of the shoe has on the heel.

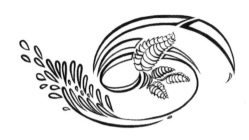

CYSTITIS

◑ Caution

---

*FOR INFORMATION RELATED TO THIS CONDI-
TION REFER TO URINARY TRACT IN THIS SECTION
- SECTION ONE.*

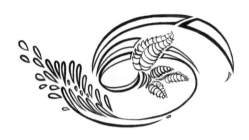

DANDRUFF

1 – Apply to the scalp the juice of a whole lemon, including peel and 50mls of water. Leave on scalp for 10 minutes then shampoo off. Final rinse with ¼ glass of lemon juice to 500mls of warm water. Let dry.

In final rinse blend ½ cup of apple cider vinegar to 1 litre of water let hair dry. This will remove the acid mantle.

2 – To assist the scalp to repair massage a good quality virgin cold-pressed olive or coconut oil to the scalp and leave on overnight. Place a towel on pillow or wear a shower cap.

◑ **Note**

*Reduce sugar and processed foods in the diet as this can cause scalp dryness.

DEPRESSION

Depression is a challenge and it requires the combination of counselling, nutrition and support, conducted within a caring, safe and secure environment. The nutritional aspects to be considered include a range of foods to include and a range of foods to avoid. The foods to avoid are highly processed foods including sugar. The foods to increase are:

1 – Introduce half an avocado into your diet.

2 – Introduce broccoli into your daily diet.

3 – Introduce lettuce juice either separately or as part of a combination of juices.

4 – Introduce apples into the diet

5 – Introduce carrot into the diet.

6 – Egg and lettuce sandwiches houses good nerve salts, protein and lecithin. A good food choice.

7 – Introduce either three fresh or dried apricots into your daily diet.

8 – Introduce rolled oats into your diet or drink oat milk. (Refer to Rolled Oats in Section Two).

9 – Introduce energy smoothies or juices (See Section Six).

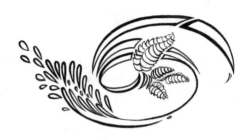

DIABETES Type 11

It is imperative that all who have diabetes are monitored by a medical practitioner, preferably a GP and an Endocrinologist. A natural medicine practitioner can also offer useful assistance and it is the blend of both fields of medicine that offers the best results.

1 – A cup of lightly steamed beans, introduced into your daily diet, can help to regulate insulin levels. Study trials have shown that late onset diabetes has been assisted by the introduction of one cup of beans daily, to the point of allowing the patient to avoid going onto insulin. The beans have been able to assist in regulating the insulin through the pancreas. This daily regime will also assist insulin dependent diabetics and lower

the requirement. It is imperative that patients on this program monitor their blood sugar levels, as the need for the insulin can drop dramatically. This information is offered by Heinerman (1987) and reported in the Indian Journal of Medical Research and further supported through research conducted by Dr. James W. Anderson MD. Professor University of Kentucky School of Medicine, and noted in Healing Foods.

2 - Add juice of green beans to other juices - blend as desired.

3 - Eat half an onion a day to support the pancreas.

4 - Introduce kiwifruit daily.

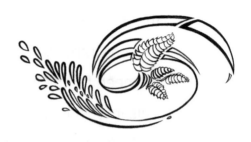

DIABETIC PERIPHERAL NEUROPATHY

This condition affects many people with diabetes.

1 - One remedy that has shown to offer good results is the introduction of GLA (gamma linolenic acid) into the diet. One source of GLA that is palatable is black currants. GLA is an omega − 6 fatty acid and the body very cleverly converts to substances that actually reduce inflammation.

2 - Add 1 cup of black current tea into the daily diet (See Section Four).

3 - Introduce fresh ginger into the diet.

4 - Introduce chilli into the diet, start slowly until you get used to it.

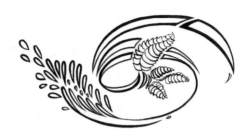

DIARRHOEA

1 – Grate two apples, including their peel, and do not eat until they have turned brown after having been exposed to the air for a short time.

2 – Eating over—ripe bananas can successfully treat this condition.

3 – Take one teaspoon of powdered blackberry root (must not have been sprayed) in a small amount of water. For much quicker results the powder may be sprinkled onto a fully ripe banana and eaten. (Refer to Blackberry in Section Two for the method used to powder the blackberry root.) It must be noted that the root of the blackberry has a strong astringent taste that draws the mouth tight and causes it to be dry and sensitive. You may find you need to drink extra fluid.

4 - Carrot can assist in preventing diarrhoea. If you have a tendency to suffer from this condition introduce carrot regularly into your diet and have a practitioner assess your diet.

5 - Eat finely sliced raw pineapple.

6 - Drink loquat leaf tea.

Infantile

1 - Give the child grated apple, with the peel.

2 - After scraping the outer layer off 500gms.of carrot, make into a soup by cutting the carrot into small pieces and boiling in one litre of water, until soft. Puree the carrot and water and add enough water to bring it back to one litre. This formula can be diluted by half if you wish to administer by bottle. For children less than three months old it is important to dilute the formula with milk. Dilute it with one part formula and two parts milk preferably goat milk or breast milk, as dairy milk may exacerbate the condition. Must be refrigerated.

Adult (with mucous or inflammation of the bowel)

1 –   Eat grated apple, with the peel.

2 –   Eat over ripe bananas.

3 –   Eat one grated apple, including the peel, combined with one grated carrot.

4 –   Eat globe artichoke to assist with bile flow.

5 –   Drink loquat leaf tea.

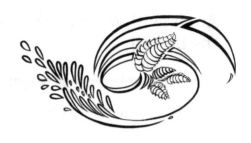

DIGESTION

To improve digestion:

1 – Eat an apple, including the peel, after a meal.

2 – Introduce globe artichoke into your diet.

3 – Raw, grated beetroot, combined with natural yogurt, will treat poor digestion.

4 – Introduce broccoli into your diet as it is particularly good for the glands of the body, especially those that aid the digestive system.

5 – Introduce cabbage into your diet as its chlorine content aids digestion.

6 – The combination of cabbage, carrot and beetroot juice promotes a very healthy breakdown of food.

7 – Young eggplant will assist with the breaking

down of protein that is difficult to digest, such as that found in most meats.

8 – Add peppermint leaves to food, in salads, or drink a cup of mint or peppermint tea 1 hour after eating (See Section Four).

9 – Grow lemon balm and have 10 leaves in a cup of herb tea. Combine with mint or peppermint or chamomile tea (See Section Four).

10 – The introduction of pawpaw into your diet will assist in the breaking down of food. Cubes of this fruit can also be used to marinate meat so as to break down the meat particles before cooking.

11 – Drinking a combination of pawpaw and pineapple juice aids in the breaking down of food.

12 – Introduce grapefruit regularly into your diet.

13 – Introduce sorrel into your diet. (Please read Sorrel in Section Two before eating it as there are some conditions in which sorrel can be harmful).

14 – Introduce kiwi fruit into your diet.

15 – Drink chamomile tea to soothe and relax the intestinal tract (See Section Four).

16 – Drink fennel tea to aid in the digestion of food (See Section Four).

17 – Drink meadowsweet tea (See Section Four).

18 – Drink potato juice to aid digestion.

GAS

1 — The relief from excessive gas, caused through slow digestion, can be gained by drinking equal parts of carrot and apple juice.

2 — Drink either fennel, mint or peppermint tea or combine them (See Section Four).

3 — Introduce fennel into the diet.

4 — Introduce pawpaw or papaya into the diet.

5 — Introduce pineapple into the diet.

6 — Drink lemon balm tea.

7 — Combine and drink meadowsweet tea and chamomile tea (See Section Four).

The need to stabilise the function of the stomach

1 — Introduce celery into your diet half an hour after food.

2 — Drink chamomile tea (See Section Four).

3 — Drink ginger and lemon tea (See Section Four).

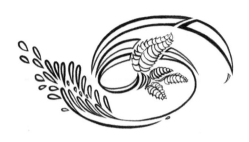

EAR ACHE

◑ Caution

---

*Before trying any treatment, consult your medical practitioner, to determine the cause of the ear ache. (Children must not have Grommet to use this formula).

---

1 – Cut half an apple, warm it and place over the ear to create an analgesic effect.

2 – Apply onion oil directly inside the ear, making sure that it is warm not hot (See Section Four).

ECZEMA

1 – Introduce five asparagus stalks into your daily diet.

2 – Introduce globe artichoke into your diet on a regular basis, particularly if your condition is due to poor diet.

3 – Eat dandelion leaves, in a green salad, to aid in elimination through bowel and liver function.

4 – Apply sweet almond oil directly to the affected area (See Section Five).

5 – Eat half an avocado every second day.

6 – Massage the area with the inner side of avocado skin (flesh removed).

7 – Drink green bean pod tea (See Section Four).

8 – Apply the undiluted juice of a whole lemon, including peel, to the condition - allow it to dry on the skin.

9 – Introduce a range of juices that support the skin and the liver (See Section Six).

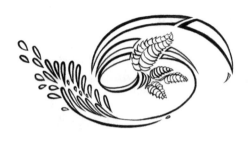

EMOTIONAL INSTABILITY

It is absolutely imperative that a professional is consulted who can guide and support, however the better you feel physically, the more energy you have the better you will feel.

1 - The introduction of corn into the diet will help to regulate the thyroid. This is particularly true when the condition is not evident in pathology reports but is unstable enough to cause emotional instability.

2 - Introduce lettuce juice into the diet as it is high in nerve salts.

3 - Ensure diet is well balanced and not high in processed foods, sugar and fats.

4 - Reduce sugar and processed foods from the diet.

Refer to anxiety in this section

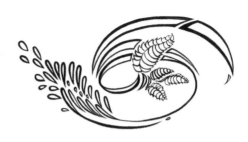

IRRITABILITY

1 – Introduce corn into your diet.

2 – Introduce lettuce juice.

3 – Eat rolled oats regularly.

4 – Ensure protein levels are adequate.

5 – Introduce a range of smoothies and juices

6 – Reduce refined sugar

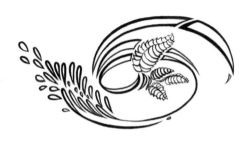

EMPHYSEMA

1 – The introduction of blackberry fruit regularly into your diet will assist with lung disease.

2 – Eat horseradish. This can be eaten as a complementary addition to a main meal.

3 – Drink a combination of the juice from half an onion and the juice of four cabbage leaves.

4 – Introduce a range of smoothies and juices into the diet (See Section Six).

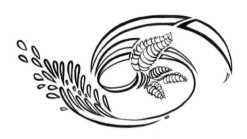

EYE TONER

1 – Chamomile tea applied onto closed eyes –

– Use thick gauze or eye pads soaked in chamomile tea. Relax and enjoy.

2 – Alternatively – Apply cucumber slices onto eyes or prepare peeled cucumber juice and blend with 50% cucumber juice with 50% chamomile tea.

3 – To an eye bath add saline solution and 2 drops of white vinegar. Wash the eyes. (Not a fruit or vegetable but too good to leave out.

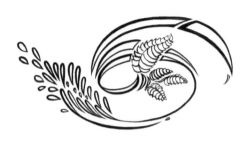

FATIGUE/LOW LEVELS OF PHYSICAL AND MENTAL ENERGY

1. Eat fifteen almonds daily (preferably roasted).
2. Drink almond milk, combined with apple juice, making sure that the peel has been juiced with the apple. (Refer to Almond in Section Two for Almond Milk Recipe.)
3. Eat dried apricots for an energy boost.
4. Drink lemon balm and/or yarrow tea (See Section Four).
5. Introduce globe artichoke into your diet, for energy throughout the day.
6. For an energy boost that will keep you going for a number of hours, eat half an avocado, with mashed almonds and finely chopped apple in the centre.

7 – Fatigue, due to over work, can be assisted with the introduction of a cup of beans into your daily diet.

8 – Carrot is an energy stimulant.

9 – Celery provides energy by stimulating the adrenal glands.

10 – Figs are an energy stimulant.

11 – Introduce sorrel into your diet. (Please read Sorrel in Section Two before eating it).

12 – Drink apple peel tea (See Section Four).

13 – Eat kiwi fruit.

14 – Introduce coriander powder or fresh herb to the diet.

15 – Reduce highly processed foods and refined sugar.

FLUID RETENTION

1 – The introduction of celery into your diet will help eliminate the retention of fluid around the body.

2 – Eat dandelion leaves as part of a daily salad.

3 – Eat horseradish. This can be eaten as a complementary addition to a main meal.

4 – Pineapple juice acts as an effective diuretic.

5 – Grapefruit also acts as an effective diuretic.

6 – Introduce watermelon into the diet as it acts as an excellent diuretic.

7 – Drink parsley tea daily. This will be particularly helpful in aiding the flushing of excess fluid that is associated with hormonal conditions (See Section Four).

8 – Drink cranberry juice daily.

9 – Wrap lightly steamed loquat leaves around the area and cover with gladwrap and leave on for a few hours.

10 – Drink loquat leaf tea (See Section Four).

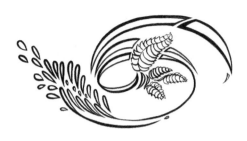

FOOD POISONING

This is a very concerning condition and one that produces pain and discomfort. At times hospitalisation is required. The key point is to allow the body to eliminate the offending food and then it is a matter of concentrating on rebuilding the body, restoring the lost nutrients.

1 – One of my all-time favourites and one that has been reported by clients to produce astounding results is black currant tea (See Section Four).

2 – Juice 1 apple, ¼ raw beetroot, 1 carrot and a handful of peppermint

3 – Make a strong peppermint tea and blend together and sip at least 3 a day to restore and settle, assisting the liver function at the same time.

4 – Introduce digestive smoothie or juices (See Section Six).

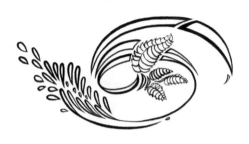

GALL BLADDER DYSFUNCTION

◑ CAUTION

Gallstones can cause a problem. Ensure you are guided by a wholistically trained health care provider.

---

1 – Introduce 15mls. of beetroot juice into your daily diet, or alternatively eat one small grated beetroot combined with natural yogurt, regularly.

2 – Drink a combination of both carrot and apple juice.

3 – Introduce globe artichoke regularly into your diet.

4 – Introduce lightly steamed cabbage into your diet.

5 – Eat barley as it is rich in insoluble fibre.

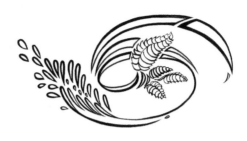

GENERAL POOR HEALTH

1 – An early European recipe that is recommended for good health is to grate one small raw beetroot, one small grated apple and about one third of a very thinly sliced cucumber with the skin on. Make a salad dressing of light olive oil, lemon juice and chopped parsley and pour over the salad.

2 – Introduce corn into your diet.

3 – Eat fresh fruits and vegetables, preferably 70% raw.

4 – Eat half an avocado every second day.

5 – The introduction of fresh pineapple juice will provide a boost to the immune system due to its high vitamin content.

6 – Eat more sprouts.

7 – Drink vegetables and fruit juices at a ratio of 3 vegetables and 1 fruit.

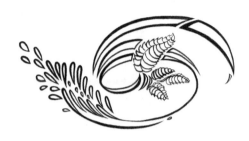

GOUT

1 - Drink 200mls.of apple juice daily, making sure that the peel has been juiced with the apple.

2 - Introduce alfalfa sprouts into your daily diet.

3 - Drink 100mls.of cherry juice daily.

4 - Introduce beans, either lightly steamed or juiced, into your daily diet.

5 - Apply a cabbage poultice or ointment, 10% juice combined with 90% Vegetable Sorbalene, (ensure vegetable based) applied to the area where there is the pain associated with gout.

6 - Introduce cauliflower into your diet.

7 - Introduce figs into your diet.

8 - Introduce globe artichoke into your diet.

9 - Introduce cucumber regularly into your diet.

10 – Drink three cups of alfalfa tea daily (See Section Four).

11 – Avoid the following:

- Alcohol
- Red meat
- Game meat
- Offal
- Fish roe
- Crustaceans.

12 – Choose foods that are high in Zinc, Vitamin C and Magnesium.

Zinc

- Almonds
- Artichokes
- Avocado
- Lettuce
- Asparagus
- Cauliflower
- Onions
- Garlic

Vitamin C

- Cherries

- Parsley
- Capsicum
- Brussel sprouts
- Lemon
- Orange
- Strawberries

Magnesium

- Bananas
- Dandelion Leaves
- Garlic
- Potatoes
- Beetroot
- Carrot
- Almonds
- Wild rice

13 - Eat ten cherries daily, or with seasonal interchange, eat five strawberries daily.

HAIR LOSS

1 – Introduce 100mls. of cucumber juice into your daily diet.

2 – Massage aloe vera gel (purchased from a health food store) into the scalp daily.

3 – When washing hair, wash with baby shampoo and rinse with a combination of half a cup of apple cider vinegar and 500mls. of water.

4 – High mineral foods will assist hair growth. Eat raw fresh fruits and vegetables.

5 – Reduce sugar and highly processed foods.

◑ **Note**

Baldness may be genetic and nothing is going to activate growth, however there are many occasions where a good diet, hair and scalp support may activate growth.

Baldness may develop due to under-lying illness — consult a health care provider.

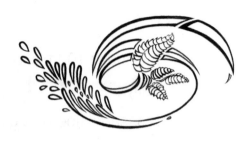

HAIR SCALP (dry)

1 – Having washed hair with a mild shampoo apply
a protein rinse:

1 egg whipped

1 tablespoon castor oil

1 tablespoon glycerine

1 teaspoon apple cider vinegar

Mix all together, leave for 15 minutes and rinse.

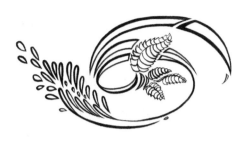

HAY FEVER

◑ Caution

A condition that produces uncomfortable symp-toms. Management must continue for at least 12 months. Hayfever and allergies may be treated with the following:

Introduce into your diet on a regular basis:

1 – Horseradish — more when condition is active.
2 – ½ bunch of watercress taken daily in salads, sandwiches or just chew.
3 – Garlic — more when condition is active.
4 – Orange peel tea — more when condition is active (See Section Four).

5 - Orange peel and honey — finely chopped orange peel and cover with honey. Have 1 teaspoon a day for prevention and up to 5 teaspoons a day when hay fever is active.

6 - Wash eyes that itch with honey and salt water, 3 drops of honey, pinch of salt water in a warm eye bath - wash eyes as often as necessary.

7 - Bananas have been reported by North Queenslanders to offer relief from hay fever by eating 1 banana a day. (look for the bananas that are round as they will taste the best).

8 - Fenugreek tea has been reported to aid in the reduction of symptoms of hay-fever (See Section Four).

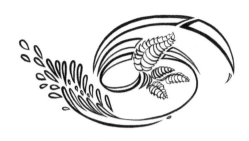

HEADACHE

1 – Eat apples, either juiced or whole, making sure that the peel is included.

2 – Apply a cabbage leaf to the forehead for relief of headaches.

3 – Drink 50mls.of lettuce juice to reduce pain.

4 – Apply a cool towel across forehead and back of neck — rest.

5 – Drink 300mls of oat milk (See Section Two).

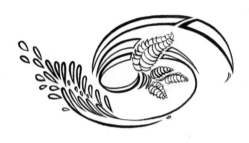

HEARTBURN

Heartburn is a very debilitating condition and one that produces exceptional pain. The following may offer assistance.

1 - Introduce oat milk into the diet.
2 - Introduce potato juice into the diet.
3 - Introduce pawpaw or papaya into the diet.
4 - Introduce a small amount of fresh pineapple into the diet.
5 - Introduce digestive smoothies and juices into the diet (See Section Six).

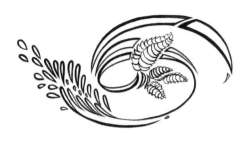

HEART HEALTH

The heart is an organ that is overlooked and only taken notice of when it malfunctions. It is a good idea to focus on this vital organ and offer medicinal foods that provide healing and support.

1 – Walnuts are a good food for the heart and the fat content is not harmful.

2 – Introduce ten dried apricot halves into your daily diet or, due to the high calorie content, a medium sized orange or banana.

3 – Introduce both onion and garlic regularly into your diet.

4 – Introduce globe artichoke into your daily diet.

5 – Introduce carrot regularly into your diet.

6 – Introduce either juiced or whole pawpaw into your diet.

7 – Introduce chillies into the diet.

8 – Introduce fresh ginger into the diet.

Palpitations

Be guided by your doctor.

1 – Boil four to five walnut shells for twenty minutes in the morning, after allowing to soak overnight. Drink three cups of this formula a day.

2 – Introduce four or five asparagus spears into your daily diet.

3 – Introduce eggplant into your daily diet.

These are all recommended as treatments but, if you are prone to this condition, then take them daily as a preventive measure.

Tired heart syndrome

1 – Introduce globe artichoke into your daily diet, combined with almond milk, to strengthen the heart.(Refer to Almond in Section Two for Almond Milk recipe).

2 – Drink hawthorn berry tea (See Section Four).

3 – Drink walnut tea (See Section Four).

4 – Follow heart health information.

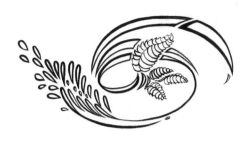

HEPATITIS

◑ Caution

Be guided by your doctor.

---

1 – Beetroot should be introduced into your diet for the treatment of all hepatitis conditions.

2 – Introduce one small, raw, grated beetroot, combined with natural yogurt, into your daily diet.

3 – Eat two apples daily.

4 – Introduce globe artichoke regularly into your diet.

5 – Introduce dandelion leaves, in salads, regularly into your diet.

6 – Drink carrot, apple and celery juices daily.

7 – Introduce green beans regularly into your diet.

8 – Eat half an avocado daily.

HERPES

◑ **Caution**

Be guided by your doctor

---

1 – Introduce apple into your daily diet, making sure that the peel is included. This is recommended as a treatment but, if you are prone to this condition, then use daily as a preventive measure.

2 – Blend 10% cabbage juice with 90% Sorbalene (purchased from the chemist), to make an ointment, and apply it to the affected area.

3 – Introduce garlic regularly into your diet.

4 – Eat dandelion leaves and calendula flowers regularly, as part of a fresh, leafy greenn salad. When herpes are active eat daily.

5 – Eliminate highly processed foods from diet and replace with fresh fruit, vegetables nuts and grains.

6 – Introduce immune supporting smoothies and juices into the diet (See Section Six).

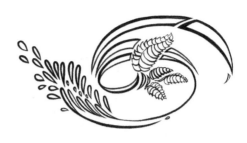

HORMONAL RELATED CONDITIONS

Sugar cravings

1 – Eat ten to fifteen almonds daily. Have one when sugar cravings occur.

Fluid retention

1 – Drink parsley tea to help the flushing of excess fluid (See Section Four).

2 – Drink celery juice or eat celery fresh.

◑ **Note**

For information on irregular bleeding and/or period pain refer to menstruation in this section - section one.

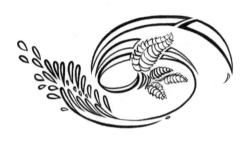

INDIGESTION

1 - Both before and after meals drink the juice of a whole lemon, including peel, and dilute it with water - 2 parts lemon to 1 part water.

2 - Drink 100mls undiluted potato juice.

3 - Introduce digestive supporting smoothies and juices into the diet (See Section Six).

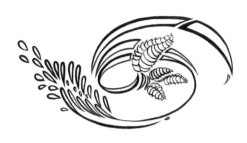

INFECTION

Recurrent in children

1 - Introduce beans into the child's diet.

2 - Introduce raw, grated carrot into the child's diet.

3 - For children 5 years and over - give 1 teaspoon of pure honey (daily).

Intestinal

1 - Introduce carrot or carrot juice, into your diet.

2 - Introduce honey if the child is 5 years of age or older - give 1 teaspoon of pure honey (dally).

3 - Introduce immune supporting juices and smoothies into the daily diet (See Section Six).

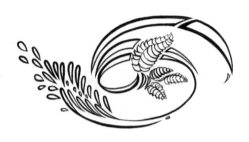

INFLAMMATION

Food can be the cause or treatment for inflammation. Foods to avoid if suffering from inflammation are:

1 - Processed sugar and highly processed foods
2 - Diet foods and drinks such as lo-cal.
3 - Watch for sensitivity to tomato, oranges and other citrus and potatoes. While some people are not sensitive to these foods others are very much affected.

Foods to include to help fight inflammation are:

1 - Pureed blackberry fruit produces an anti-inflammatory action and in fact, one of the compounds that is found in blackberries. This is where Brufen was derived from.

2 – Introduce raw carrots into the diet.

3 – Introduce celery in to the diet.

4 – Introduce turmeric into the diet.

5 – Introduce ginger into the diet.

6 – Introduce cloves (in tea)into the diet
(See Section Four).

7 – Introduce apples into the diet.

8 – Introduce cinnamon into the diet.

9 – Introduce blueberries into the diet.

10 – Introduce black current tea (See Section Four).

11 – Introduce avocado into the diet

12 – Introduce cherries into the diet.

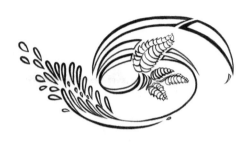

INFLUENZA (COLDS, FLU)

1 – Apple fast for three days. The apples can be prepared in any variety of ways, making sure that the peel is always included.

2 – Drinking beetroot juice was a remedy prescribed by early physicians for the treatment of influenza. (This is not recommended for diabetics because of the high sugar content). This juice is particularly effective in dealing with this condition if combined with apple juice.

3 – Add a pinch of cayenne powder, (available at supermarkets) to a small amount of water and take this preparation a couple of times a day.

4 – Apple peel tea (See Section Four).

5 – Lemon balm tea (See Section Four).

6 - Yarrow tea consumed throughout the day is of benefit.

7 - Radish (3) and (1) apple juiced.

8 - Cinnamon tea (See Section Four)

9 - Introduce immune smoothies and juices into the daily diet (See Section Six).

◑ **Note**

---

*must stay indoors and warm

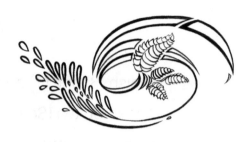

COUGHING

1 - Drink almond milk (See Section Two).

2 - Drink onion and honey syrup (See Section Two).

3 - Radish, apple and clove. Juice radish (3) and (1) apple and a pinch of powdered clove.

4 - Introduce immune smoothies and juices (See Section Six).

5 - Introduce horseradish into the diet.

6 - Introduce yarrow and peppermint or mint tea into the diet (See Section Four).

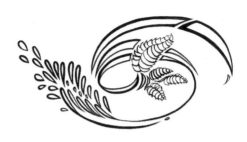

INSECT BITES

Important to apply first aid to bite and consider removal of sting, then:

1 – Apply the juice of a whole lemon to the area.
2 – Apply vegemite to bite as a fast pain reliever. (Not a fruit or vegetable but too affective to leave out).
3 – Apply toothpaste to the area, seems any brand works.
4 – Apply Apple cider vinegar to the bite.
5 – Apply a slice of raw potato to the sting.
6 – Apply mashed pawpaw or papaya to the area.

Reaction to insect bites

Seek medical advice and:

1 – Bee sting - onion poultice to draw sting.
2 – Wasp - ice or onion poultice.
3 – Mosquito - Apply lavender oil directly onto the bite.
   – Apply tea tree oil directly onto the bite.
   – Apply eucalyptus oil directly onto the bite.
   – Apply vegemite to bite.
   – Introduce apples into your diet - juiced or whole, making sure that the peel is included as they are packed with Vitamin B group and mossies do not like that!
   – Drink apple cider vinegar and lemon drink daily to purify the blood.
   – 10mls of apple cider vinegar to the juice of 1 lemon and water to dilute (to taste).

INSOMNIA

1 – Drink warmed apple juice nightly, making sure that the peel is included.

2 – Drink a small glass of celery juice just prior to retiring for the night.

3 – Drink chamomile tea just prior to retiring for the night. (ensure it is a strong infusion).

4 – Eat foods high in calcium.

5 – Eat an apple 30 minutes before bed.

6 – Eat ½ banana 30 minutes before bed.

7 – Add cherries to the diet. Although a short season freeze when in season. Have 12 cherries 30minutes before bed or 1 glass of cherry juice. Due to nutrient rich and melatonin source they may assist.

8 – (Often the body's bio—rhythm needs resetting — skip one nights' sleep and this will often reset the rhythm).

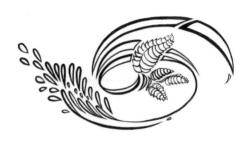

IRON – low

Many conditions develop due to low iron. These range from tiredness to split nails and many in-between. Make sure your practitioner checks your iron levels and if low the following may be of assistance.

1 – Mushrooms
2 – Apricots (dried)
3 – Dark leafy greens
4 – Watercress
5 – Sun dried tomatoes
6 – Parsley
7 – Olives

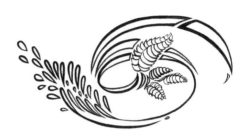

IRRITABILITY

1 – Introduce corn into your diet.

2 – Eat more uncooked fresh fruit and vegetables.

3 – Eat Vitamin B6 foods, such as pineapple,
     walnuts, sunflower seeds and oats.

4 – Drink lettuce juice.

5 – Introduce rolled oats into the diet.

6 – Introduce apples into the diet.

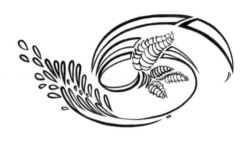

IRRITABLE COLON

1 - Introduce grated apple into your daily diet, making sure that the peel is included. This is recommended as a treatment but, if you are prone to this condition, then take it daily as a preventive measure.

2 - Eat very ripe bananas.

3 - Combine grated carrot and grated apple into the diet and add a small amount of apple cider vinegar.

4 - Drink slippery elm tea three times a day (See Section Four).

5 - Ensure the flora is balanced by including a good quality natural yoghurt.

6 - Introduce digestive smoothies and juices (See Section Six).

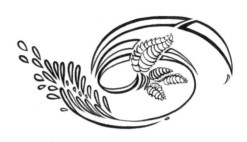

KIDNEY CONDITIONS

Pain relief

1 – Application of a cabbage leaf to the back, over the kidney region, will help with pain relief.

2 – Drink corn silk tea (See Section Four).

3 – Drink couch-grass tea (See Section Four).

Promoting normal kidney function

1 – Introduce asparagus into your diet. Important note: It is imperative that there is no inflammation of the kidney as this will be aggravated by the asparagus.

2 – When wanting to support any urinary tract problem or infection, introduce cauliflower into your diet. Combine this with dandelion leaf salad.

3 – Introducing celery regularly into your diet helps promotes normal kidney function.

4 – The introduction of horseradish into your diet will assist the function of the kidney.

5 – Drink one glass of barley water, three times a day. (Barley water can be purchased from the super market or alternatively soak barley overnight in water and strain).

6 – Introduce watermelon regularly into your diet.

7 – Drink corn silk tea (See Section Four).

8 – Drink couch-grass tea (See Section Four).

Stones

◐ **Caution**

It is important to note that this is meant as a complementary formula and should be taken in conjunction with those medicines prescribed by your medical practitioner.

– Bean juice helps to eliminate small kidney stones.

– Drink corn silk tea (See Section Four).

LACTATION

To decrease

1 – Introduce globe artichoke into your daily diet. This will result in your milk supply totally drying up.

To promote

1 – Cover fifteen almonds with barley water and puree it. Drink this formula to produce a more nutritious milk. (Barley water can be purchased from the super market or alternatively soak barley overnight in water and strain).

2 – European studies have shown that the substitution of almond milk for breast milk has proven to be very successful (See Section Two).

3 – To increase the flow of breast milk place cabbage leaves over the breasts and they will act as a drawing agent on the milk.

4 – Introduce carrot into your diet.

5 – Drink aniseed tea (See Section Four).

6 – Drink fenugreek tea (See Section Four).

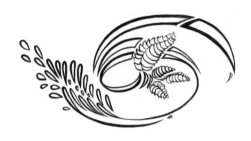

LARYNGITIS

1 - Gargle warmed carrot juice.

2 - Gargle a quarter of a teaspoon of cayenne powder in half a cup of warm water.

3 - Drink sage tea (See Section Four).

4 - Introduce apple and radish juice.

5 - Introduce black currants that have been soaked in apple cider vinegar diluted with 50% water. Eat the currants and consume some of the liquid in small teaspoon doses.

6 - Introduce watercress, parsley, onion, lemon, ginger and clove juice (See Section Six).

7 - Introduce immune and blood purifying smoothies and juices into the diet (See Section Six).

LIBIDO - LOW

1 – Russian research shows that avocado is a sexual stimulant. This is recommended as a treatment but, if you are prone to this condition, then eat avocado regularly as a preventive measure.

2 – Introduce celery regularly into your diet as the mineral and vitamin matrix that comes into the system, via the celery, is favourable to energy production, particularly of a sexual nature.

3 – Drink hops as a tea to assist in the elevation of a woman's libido (See Section Four).

4 – The drinking of a teaspoon of chopped parsley to a cup of hot water will assist in increasing the libido of both men and women.

◑ **Note**

Psychological issues may need addressing and a trained counsellor can be of assistance.

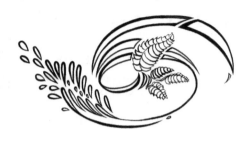

LIVER DISORDERS

1 – Drink apple juice daily, making sure that the peel is juiced with the apple.

2 – Introduce globe artichoke regularly into your diet.

3 – Introduce 30mls. of beetroot juice into your diet.

4 – Eat calendula flowers and dandelion leaves in salads.

5 – Drink twice daily a combination formula of the juice of one carrot, one apple and 45mls. of celery juice.

6 – Combine 2 tablespoons of apple cider vinegar.

7 – Drink loquat leaf tea (See Section Four).

Liver cell regeneration

1 – Eat dandelion leaves in green salads.

2 – Eat two apples daily.

3 – When in season, introduce watermelon regularly into your diet.

4 – Drink a mixture of globe artichoke in liquid formulation, as prescribed by herbalists, combined with apple juice. This will result in better liver function.

5 – Introduce beans into your daily diet.

6 – Reduce highly processed foods and increase fresh fruits, vegetables, nuts and grains.

7 – Drink loquat leaf tea (See Section Four).

8 – Introduce beetroot into the diet.

Liver and de-tox help

1 – Take globe artichoke in a liquid formulation, as prescribed by herbalists.

2 – Introduce globe artichoke regularly into the diet.

3 – Drink dandelion root tea (See Section Four).

4 – Drink combination vegetable juices as they are beneficial in reducing toxins.

5 – Introduce loquats into the diet.

6 – Drink loquat leaf tea (See Section Four).

7 – Introduce a range of sprouts (all are good for you).

8 – Introduce broccoli into the diet.

9 – Introduce a range of smoothies and juices to support liver (See Section Six).

Liver and increase bile flow

1 – Introduce globe artichoke into your daily diet.

2 – Introduce cabbage into your diet.

3 – Eat dandelion leaves in green salads.

4 – Drink pure lemon juice ensuring the peel is included.

5 – Drink 2 tablespoons of apple cider vinegar combined with the juice of 1 lemon (including the peel) and 1 teaspoon of honey to 50mls of water.

6 – Introduce all leafy greens in particular the outer dark bitter leaves.

7 – Introduce liver support smoothies and juices to the diet (See Section Six).

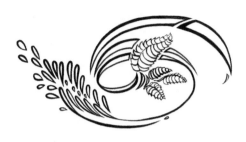

LUMBAGO

1 - Apply a cabbage poultice to the lower back.

2 - Apply a poultice of castor oil to the lower back.

3 - Eat blackcurrants soaked in water overnight and drink liquid.

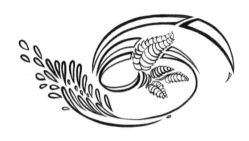

MOUTH ULCERS

1 – Carrot and watercress juice offers good results. Simply juice 1 whole carrot including the tops if available and a good handful of watercress.

2 – Watercress juice approximately 50mls

3 – Combine a handful of coriander and a handful of watercress, juice and drink.

4 – Introduce immune smoothies and juices into the diet (See Section Six).

5 – Introduce cloves into the daily diet in the form of tea or added to smoothies or juices.

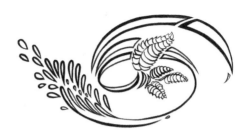

MENSTRUATION

Cramps

1 – Warmed blackberry juice or blackberry tea made with the leaves, has an anti- spasm effect. (Refer to Section Four for Blackberry Tea).

2 – Drink dried parsley tea (See Section Four).

3 – Drink hot ginger tea (See Section Four).

4 – Apply castor oil poultice to the abdomen.

Irregularity

1 – Introduce the whole blackberry plant (root, leaf and fruit) into the diet (See Section Two).

2 – Drink caraway seed tea (See Section Four).

3 – Drink dried parsley and/or sage tea regularly,

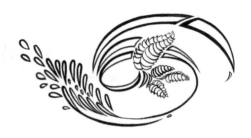

MIGRAINES

Assuming that the condition has been professionally diagnosed, the successful management for migraines is to find the therapy that is right for you. Some of the therapies are:

1 - Take one teaspoon of apple cider vinegar (purchased from a super market or health food store) daily. This supplies multi minerals that assist the blood vessels to function normally. It is important to note the apple cider vinegar must be naturally fermented. This will be stated on the label.

2 - Eat two leaves of feverfew plant daily. This plant may be grown or alternatively, capsules (purchased from a health food store), be taken daily.

3 – The common condition of allergic migraines presents when the body cannot cope with a food that has been consumed. Include a bitter salad combination as a pre-meal snack.

4 – Wrap a cold towel around the head. Sit and rest for 30 minutes.

5 – Ensure neck muscles are supple. Employ regular massage therapy.

6 – Drink oatmilk regularly (See Section Four).

◑ **Note**

All the therapies that have any success are all ongoing as a daily formula. The system must be strengthened to combat this very troublesome condition.

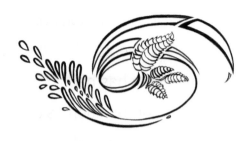

MOTION SICKNESS

1 – Avoid drinking too much fluid prior to journey but ginger tea and/or peppermint or mint tea will help to settle the stomach (See Section Four).

2 – Eat an apple and a dry piece of bread, no butter, to soak up the fluids, prior to departure and during the journey.

3 – Grate fresh ginger (one teaspoon) and add a cup of boiling water. Steep for a few minutes and sip very slowly.

4 – Deep slow breathing in the nose and out the mouth, preferably closing the eyes.

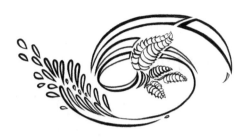

MUSCLE HEALTH

1 – Eat three apricots daily, preferably fresh.

2 – Introduce broccoli into your diet.

3 – Eat fresh, raw fruit and vegetables.

4 – Introduce avocados into the diet.

5 – Eat fully ripened bananas.

Muscle aches

1 – Introduce leafy green salads into the daily diet.

2 – Remove all low calorie foods and drinks from your diet as these may produce muscle pain.

3 – Introduce muscle health smoothies and juices into the diet (See Section Six).

4 – Use cayenne lotion to massage the affected area (See Section Two).

5 – Use cool towels or ice packs.

6 – Refer to inflammation in this section.

NAILS

Ridging

1 - Eat half an avocado twice a week, for six weeks, as part of a meal or by itself.

2 - Eat an increased amount of leafy green salad.

3 - Reduce highly processed foods - increase fresh fruit and vegetables.

4 - Massage almond meal and sorbalene cream into nails.

    a - 1 teaspoon of almond meal and 3 teaspoons of sorbalene combined.

5 - Eat iron rich foods (See Low Iron).

Splitting

1 - Due to its high mineral content, drinking a wine glass of cucumber juice daily, will assist recovery from this condition.

2 - Drink a combination of freshly squeezed vegetable juices.

3 - Eat bananas.

4 - Eat avocados.

5 - Reduce refined sugar and ensure good hydration by sipping water throughout the day.

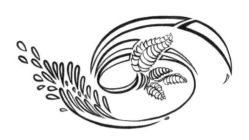

NAPPY RASH

1 – Change nappies regularly and apply chickweed ointment (purchased at the health food store) with each change.

2 – Apply almond oil lightly after bathing and then chickweed ointment (purchased at the health food store) (See Section Five).

Urine scalding

1 – Give the baby a small amount of corn silk tea. This is quite palatable for the baby and will decrease the concentration of urine (See Section Four).

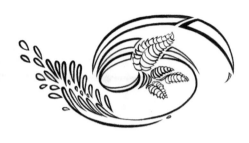

NAUSEA

Nausea can occur for many reasons and can be quite debilitating. Old fashioned remedies offer solutions.

1 - Drink pineapple juice by sipping small amounts regularly.

2 - Grated ginger in a small amount of water or blended into pineapple juice.

3 - Lemon and sugar water by mixing the juice of 2 lemons and 3 teaspoons of sugar or honey. Take by the teaspoon.

4 - Introduce digestive smoothies or juices (See Section Six).

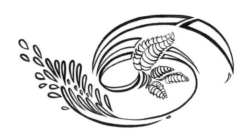

NIGHT BLINDNESS

One of the ways of assisting eye health is to focus on bringing in health giving nutrients on a daily basis and keep the circulation moving through gentle and consistent exercise.

1 – Introduce carrot regularly into your diet.
2 – Introduce carrot, apple and bean juice into the diet (See Section Six).
3 – Introduce bilberries into the diet.
4 – Introduce ginger into the diet.
5 – Introduce berries into diet.

PAIN CONTROL (AN ANALGESIC)

1 – Drink apple juice, making sure that the peel is juiced with the apple.
2 – Eat raw lettuce.
3 – Eat raw beans.
4 – Apply a lettuce or a cabbage poultice to the area.

Pain in the joints

1 – Remove all low calorie foods and drinks from your diet.
2 – Apply a cabbage poultice over the joint.
3 – Eat an increased amount of leafy green salad.
4 – Eat fresh food and remove all processed food from your diet.
5 – Drink celery juice daily. Drink 100mls of celery juice, combined with the juice of any other preferred vegetables.
6 – Massage muscle oil blends to the affected area (See Section Five).
7 – Drink meadowsweet tea three times a day (See Section Four).
8 – Drink 1 tsp. of apple cider vinegar and the juice of ½ lemon juiced daily.
9 – Refer to inflammation in this section.

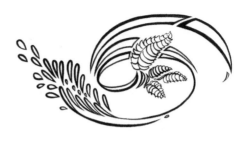

PERIODS

◑ Note

---

*FOR INFORMATION ON THIS CONDITION REFER
TO MENSTRUATION IN THIS SECTION - SECTION
ONE

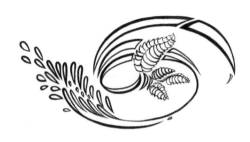

PREGNANCY

Morning sickness

1 – Beetroot is a great formulation for morning sickness. Grate raw or lightly steamed beetroot and combine it with natural yogurt.

2 – Drink strong raspberry leaf tea (See Section Four).

3 – Drink mild ginger tea (See Section Four).

4 – Eat small regular meals of fresh un-processed foods.

5 – Reduce highly processed foods.

6 – Reduce fatty foods.

7 – Reduce highly sweetened foods.

8 – Do not get hungry as this can activate morning sickness. Snack small amounts and often.

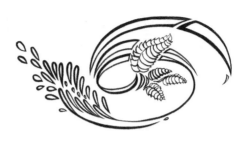

RESPIRATORY PROBLEMS

Excessive mucous

1 – Warmed carrot juice will help to breakdown the congestion that can settle on the respiratory centre.

2 – Pineapple juice can also aid with the breaking down of mucous.

3 – Introduce garlic and onion into your diet.

4 – Due to its medicinal actions, as a plant anti-biotic, the introduction of horseradish into your diet will assist with this condition. Horseradish can be eaten as a complementary addition to a main meal.

5 – Sip onion and honey syrup (See Section Four).

6 – Introduce fresh pineapple and ginger juice.

7 – Introduce radish and apple juice.

8 – Introduce radish and cabbage juice.

RESTLESS LEGS

1 - Drink a small amount of celery juice every day. Do not take yourself off this treatment too rapidly as it has been reported that this makes the condition worse.

2 - Eat an increased amount of leafy green salad.

3 - Introduce lightly steamed, leafy green vegetables into your diet.

4 - Drink turnip, carrot and lettuce juice.

5 - Drink freshly prepared vegetable juices daily to elevate mineral levels in the blood stream.

6 - Introduce coriander into the diet in powdered form or fresh leaves.

7 - Exercise legs by walking daily for 15 - 30 minutes.

8 - Reduce sugar and highly processed foods and any low-calorie foods.

9 - Ensure good hydration by sipping water regularly throughout the day.

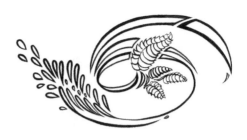

RETARDED GROWTH

Children

1 – Introduce fully ripened bananas into the child's daily diet.

2 – Consume fresh fruit and vegetables - reduce processed foods.

3 – Introduce grated carrot into daily diet.

4 – Remove refined sugar watching for cordials and soft drinks

5 – Introduce a range of smoothies and juices into the daily diet (See Section Six).

RHEUMATISM

1 - Introduce green beans, either lightly steamed or juiced, into the diet.

2 - Drink 50mls. of cabbage juice daily.

3 - An old treatment for rheumatic fingers was to apply a warmed carrot poultice to the fingers. This still works today!

4 - Introduce figs into the diet.

5 - Eat two apples, including the peel, daily.

6 - Introduce cucumber regularly into the diet.

7 - Drink celery juice regularly.

8 - Drink the combined juices of lettuce, celery, carrot and apple.

9 - Drink one tsp. of apple cider vinegar and the juice of ½ lemon daily.

10 - Ensure fluid intake is adequate say 1 litre of water a day and sip across the day.

11 - Introduce coriander powder or fresh leaves into the diet.

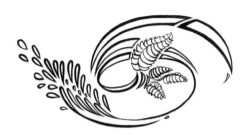

RING WORM

◑ Caution

Seek doctor's diagnosis.

---

1 – Apply a poultice of pulped apple to the affected area.

2 – Apply mashed apple and ripe banana peel to the ring worm. Wrap in gauze lightly bandage, changing the dressing daily. Maintain this routine until the condition clears.

3 – Apply a poultice of cabbage leaves to the area or apply cabbage ointment (See Section Five).

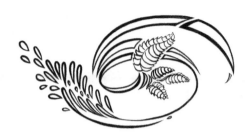

SHINGLES

1 – Apply a cabbage poultice directly over the shingles as a soothing anti-inflammatory agent.

2 – Apply cabbage ointment (See Section Five).

3 – Apply neat apple cider vinegar regularly to the area.

4 – Introduce cabbage, carrot and apple juice to the diet.

5 – Introduce lettuce and carrot juice to the diet.

6 – Introduce immune smoothies and juices to the diet (See Section Six).

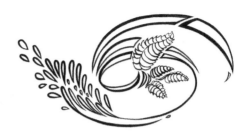

SINUS CONGESTION

1 – Blackberries, sprinkled with honey, will assist in decreasing the problems related to sinus.

2 – Eat horseradish.

3 – Wash out nasal passages with salt water wash

4 – Take 2 handfuls of eucalyptus leaves, cover with cold water place in a pot. Bring to boil and then reduce to a simmer. Breathe in the aromatics.

5 – Introduce immune smoothies and juices (See Section Six).

◑ **Note**

FOR MORE INFORMATION ON THIS CONDITION ALSO REFER TO CATARRH AND BRONCHITIS IN THIS SECTION - SECTION ONE

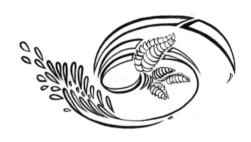

SKIN CONDITIONS

Acne

1 - Introduce avocado into your diet.

2 - Apply cabbage juice to the affected area.

3 - Drink green bean pod tea (See Section Four).

4 - Eat a balanced diet, reducing highly processed foods.

5 - Drink carrot and celery juice.

6 - Apply lemon juice (whole lemon including peel) and allow to dry.

7 - Apply lavender oil to lesions - do not squeeze them.

8 - Apply potato juice to skin to cleanse, heal, nourish and tone, (peel potato).

Acne due to poor diet

1 – Increase water intake to 2 litres per day. Sip across the day.
2 – Introduce globe artichoke regularly into your diet.
3 – Reduce highly processed foods and replace with fresh fruit, vegetables, nuts and grains.
4 – Reduce soft drinks and cordial.

Bad complexion

1 – A combination of cauliflower and carrot juice may create a healthy, clear complexion.
2 – Eat half an avocado every second day.
3 – Consume combination of vegetable juices. Select any, but ensure leafy green vegetables are included.
4 – Potato juice applied as a cleanser, (peel potato).
5 – Wash face with cold water and wipe the face with the inner skin of an avocado.

Black heads

1 – Dab apple cider vinegar onto black head.
2 – Massage lemon juice into the area and allow it to dry overnight.
3 – Dab neat lavender oil onto black head.

Burns

1 - Apply apple cider vinegar (purchased from the supermarket) to the affected area.

2 - Apply almond milk immediately, by bathing the affected area (See Section Two).

3 - Apply honey directly to the burn.

4 - Apply blended radish and ice cubes to the burnt area.

5 - Apply grated, raw potato to the affected area.

6 - Apply grated, raw pumpkin to the affected area.

7 - Apply non-diluted, pure lavender oil to the affected area (See Section Five).

Burns - skin repair

1 - Avocado oil has been known to support collagen, which is what makes the skin stick together. Every day, over a period of six days, massage avocado oil into a test area of the burn and if there is a change in the condition of the skin use it over the whole of the affected area (See Section Five).

2 - Apply lavender oil directly onto the affected area (See Section Five).

3 - Apply watercress juice to affected area.

Chaffed/dry

1 - Apply almond milk regularly by bathing the affected area until condition clears (See Section Two).

2 - Apply sweet almond oil externally to severely affected areas. This can be applied as often as is needed until condition clears (See Section Five).

3 - Apply mashed avocado to soothe the skin.

4 - Apply chickweed ointment. (Purchase from your local health food store).

5 - Massage pure honey into skin, leave on for a few minutes, then rinse off with cold water.

6 - Blend 1 tablespoon of honey to 100mls of potato water and apply.

Damaged skin

1 - Celery juice promotes the healing of damaged skin when applied externally.

2 - Apply mashed avocado directly onto the skin. Wrap in gauze or lightly bandage for protection, if needed.

3 - Drink radish juice diluted with equal parts of water. This will help to regenerate the skin.

4 - Apply potato juice to skin.

5 - Apply chickweed ointment. (Purchase from your local health food store).

6 - Massage pure honey into skin, leave on for a few minutes, then rinse off with cold water.

Dry, scaly

1 - Introduce avocado into your diet to give a smooth healthy glow to the skin.

2 - Apply sweet almond oil directly onto the affected area (See Section Five).

3 - Apply chickweed ointment. (Purchase from your local health food store).

4 - Massage pure honey into skin, leave on for a few minutes, then rinse off with cold water.

5 - Massage skin with the inside peel of avocado.

Facial neuralgia (nerve pain of the face)

1 - Apply a poultice of avocado onto the affected area.

2 - Apply hypericum ointment to affected area.

3 - Apply a castor oil poultice to affected area.

Facial steams - (cleanser)

1 – To cleanse and prepare the skin for repair a facial steam using dried chamomile flowers is exceptional.
Simply take 2 tablespoons of fresh or 1 tablespoon of dried herb or 6 teabags.
Place in a bowl of boiling water.
Place towel over head to form an enclosure for steam and feel the gentle cleanse.

Facial steams — (stimulator/toning)

6 peppermint teabags or 2 tablespoons of fresh or 1 tablespoon of dried peppermint.

Inflammation

1 – Apply almond milk regularly by bathing the affected area until condition clears (See Section Two).

Itching

1 – Apply aloe vera gel to the area. (Purchase from your local health food store).

2 – Apply cucumber juice directly to the affected area.

3 - Apply lavender oil to the affected area. (Purchase from your local health food store).

4 - Apply chickweed ointment to affected area (purchase from health food store).

5 - Combine half cucumber including peel and blend with carrot juice to equal parts.

Promoting elimination via the skin by increasing perspiration

1 - Introduce globe artichokes into your diet.

2 - Drink peppermint tea (See Section Four).

3 - Drink yarrow tea (See Section Four).

SMELLY FEET

1. Bathe the feet in warm water and add half a cup of epsom salts (purchased from a super market) and ten drops of lavender oil daily. After the bath scrub the feet thoroughly with a brush to remove dead skin layers allowing the feet to breathe (See Section Five).

2. Remove dairy products from the diet as these may be affecting the digestive system and be responsible for constipation, that in turn, may be part of the problem.

3. Eat two apples daily, remembering to include the skin.

4. Only wear good leather shoes that can air the feet.

5. Walk barefoot as often as possible, preferably on sand, as this massages the feet and removes the dead cell layer.

6. Bathe the feet in warm water with 100mls of apple cider vinegar.

7. Ensure socks are cotton or wool — never nylon or synthetic.

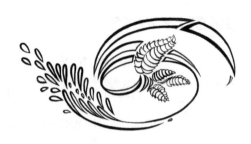

SPASM AND/OR INFLAMMATION OF THE STOMACH

1 - Drink almond milk (See Section Two).

2 - Drink camomile tea (See Section Four).

3 - Drink meadowsweet tea (See Section Four).

4 - Eat raw honey regularly.

5 - Pound carrot seeds to a powder to make up 1 teaspoon. Add to 100mls of cold water and drink.

6 - Eat black currants that have been soaked overnight in water.

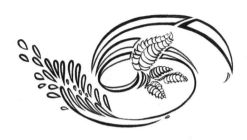

STRESS

1 - Introduce kiwi fruit regularly into your diet.

2 - Introduce rolled oats to the diet.

3 - Drink oat milk daily (See Section Two).

4 - Ensure diet is high in protein and low in fat

5 - Introduce smoothies and juices into the daily diet (See Section Six).

6 - Avoid comfort eating of foods highly processed especially sugar and fats.

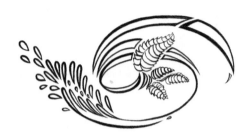

STYES

1 – Gently apply carrot oil onto the condition. This oil is a very powerful healer and will aid rapid healing (See Section Five).

2 – Recurring styes are usually an indication of poor nutrition and or a compromised immune system. Introduce immune smoothies or juices into the diet (See Section Six).

3 – Introduce carrots into the daily diet.

4 – Bathe the eyes in saline water and add 2 drops of white vinegar (not a fruit or vegetable but too good to leave out).

SUGAR CRAVINGS

Sugar cravings can be quite destructive to wellbeing as sugar is a nasty substance. One way to help reduce the cravings is to balance the diet by increasing high protein low fat foods.

Start the day with a good protein such as a boiled egg or omelette. That is a great start. Then introduce the following:

1 – Eat ten to fifteen almonds daily (preferably roasted).
2 – Consume a combination of vegetable juices daily.
3 – Eat mushrooms or green beans daily.
4 – Eat loquats when in season.
5 – Consume loquat leaf tea (See Section Four).
6 – Increase low fat proteins into the diet and reduce simple carbohydrates such as white flour produces and sugar.

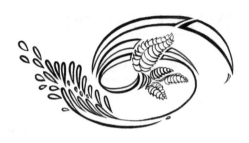

THROAT CONDITIONS

Excess mucous

1 – The pulp of the blackberry works well for this condition.

2 – Blend the juice of one lemon plus peel to two tablespoons of pure honey. Take by the teaspoon.

3 – Onion and garlic soup will help retard this condition and stimulate the immune system (See Section Two).

4 – Eat pure honey.

5 – Blend 5 loquats (whole) with 2 loquat leaves that have been air dried and the fur removed and add 1 tablespoon of honey. Take by the teaspoon.

6 – Introduce apple and radish juice.

Inflammation and/or spasms of the throat and respiratory system

1 – Drink almond milk, with the combination of half barley water and half almond puree. (Refer to Almond in Section Two for Almond Milk Recipe. Barley water can be purchased from the super market or alternatively soak barley overnight in water and strain).

2 – Eat pure honey.

3 – Blend 5 loquats (whole) with 2 loquat leaves that have been air dried and the fur removed and add 1 tablespoon of honey. Take by the teaspoon.

Sore throat

1 – Puree blackberry fruit and swallow. The Vitamins C and A and the Isocitric Acid will assist this condition. Warm the pulp just a little to avoid the tissue tightening up.

2 – Place the leaves of the blackberry into boiling water and then gargle with the preparation.

3 – Soak three dried figs in a cup of water overnight. In the morning eat the figs and drink the juice.

4 – Drinking pineapple juice can help relieve the pain of a sore throat.

5 – Drink thyme tea (See Section Four).

6 – Gargle with ¼ cup of warm water and ¼ teaspoon of black or red pepper. (Do not swallow).

7 – Blend 5 loquats (whole) with 2 loquat leaves that have been air dried and the fur removed and add 1 tablespoon of honey. Take by the teaspoon.

8 – Introduce radish and apple juice.

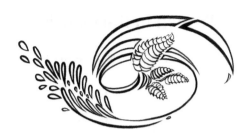

THRUSH

1 - Eat natural yogurt with acidophilus.

2 - Introduce garlic into your diet. Eat calendula flowers in leafy green salads.

3 - Introduce avocado into your daily diet whilst condition exists. If you are prone to this condition then introduce avocado regularly into your diet as a preventive treatment.

4 - Eating over ripe bananas will help with this condition.

5 - Remove all yeast foods from diet such as bread, mushrooms and pickled foods.

6 - As a vaginal douche: mix 1 part lemon juice to 5 parts water. Avoid if vaginal area is painful and use apple cider vinegar instead.

7 - Add apple cider vinegar to a bath.

*see also vaginal thrush

Thrush in the mouth

1 – Rinse the mouth with cucumber and carrot juice.

2 – Rinse your mouth with apple cider vinegar (purchased from the super market).

3 – Eat natural yogurt with acidophilus.

4 – Rinse mouth with one teaspoon of honey, one lemon juiced (plus peel), and warm water **(Do not swallow).**

TINEA

Mild cases

1 - Apply tea tree oil topically to the affected area. This can be applied as often as needed until condition clears (See Section Five).

2 - All socks and stocking should be washed in hot soapy water and in the final rinse add twenty drops of tea tree oil (See Section Five).

3 - Apply thyme oil (See Section Five).

Stubborn cases

1 - Use the pulp of one avocado, with 10 drops of thyme oil added. Apply and leave on overnight. This should be repeated nightly until condition clears.
(Refer to Section Five for information regarding Thyme Oil).

2 - Apply carrot oil to affected area (See Section Five).

3 - All shoes should be aired outdoors.

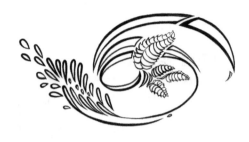

TIRED LEG SYNDROME

1 - This condition may respond to a small amount of celery juice taken daily.

2 - Take combined vegetable juices daily to increase mineral content in the blood.

3 - Increase magnesium rich foods.

◑ **Note**

⋆refer restless legs in this section.

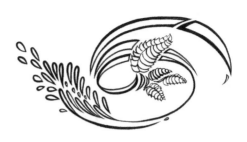

TISSUE FIRMING –

Face, neck, breasts, abdomen and the wrinkling associated with post pregnancy.

1 – Using freshly squeezed apple juice, making sure the peel is juiced with the apple, massage into area you wish to treat. Leave on.

2 – Apply aloe vera gel to the area. (Purchase from your local health food store).

3 – Combine ½ apple juice with ½ aloe vera juice and massage into the affected area. Leave on.

TONSILITIS

◐ **Caution**

It is important to note that this is meant as a complementary formula and should be taken in conjunction with those medicines prescribed by your medical practitioner.

---

1 − Drink almond milk. This preparation is recommended as a treatment but, if you are prone to this condition, then drink it daily as a preventive measure (See Section Two).

2 − Gargle with warmed carrot juice.

3 − Gargle with $\frac{1}{8}$th tsp. of cayenne pepper in half a glass of warm water, with a pinch of salt added.

4 − Gargle freshly squeezed whole lemon juice, including peel.

5 − Gargle 30mls of freshly squeezed whole lemon with 2 crushed or powdered cloves.

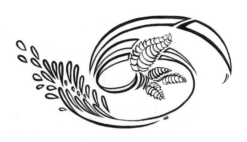

TOXAEMIA

1 – Introduce broccoli into your diet.

Consider introducing products from the following list.

Toxin release from the body - assisting with

1 – Drink apple peel tea daily (See Section Four).

2 – Introduce globe artichoke into your daily diet.

3 – Introduce four or five stalks of asparagus into your daily diet for the elimination of toxins from all eliminating organs, including the scalp.

4 – Introduce cabbage regularly into your diet.

5 – Celery helps to eliminate toxic waste from the body.

6 – Eliminate heavy, processed foods from your diet.

7 – Increase the amount of leafy green vegetables in your diet. These may be juiced or steamed.

8 - Alfalfa sprouts help to eliminate toxic waste from the body.

9 - Eat grated, raw beetroot three times a week.

10 - Drink apple cider vinegar - 2 tablespoons in a small amount of water consumed daily.

◑ **Note**

FOR FURTHER INFORMATION RELATED TO THIS CONDITION REFER TO TOXINS IN THIS SECTION - SECTION ONE.

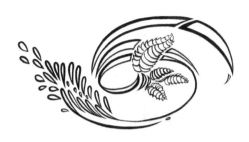

ULCERS IN THE DIGESTIVE SYSTEM

1 - Introduce figs into your diet.

2 - Drink 200mls.of cabbage juice daily.

3 - Drink meadowsweet tea (See Section Four).

4 - Eat pure honey regularly.

5 - Juice cabbage to make 200mls of cabbage juice, add 1 tablespoon of honey and ¼ teaspoon of bi-carb.

Ulcers in the mouth

1 - Rinse the mouth with carrot and cucumber juice.

2 - Rinse mouth with cabbage juice and then swallow.

3 - Rinse mouth with diluted whole lemon juice, including the peel.

4 - Take honey into mouth and hold on the area, then swallow.

5 - Watercress juiced.

6 - Rinse mouth with 30mls of cabbage juice and 1 tsp. of honey. Repeat up to 3 times a day.

Ulcers in the stomach

1 - Drink 200mls.of cabbage juice twice daily.

2 - Drink the juice of one potato, combined with the juice often cabbage leaves, twice daily.

3 - Introduce mashed pumpkin regularly into your diet.

4 - Drink meadowsweet tea twice daily (See Section Four).

5 - Eat pure honey regularly.

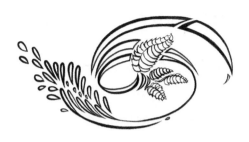

URINARY TRACT - *Gravel In The Urine*

1 - Introduce cucumber regularly into your diet.

2 - Drink three cups of corn silk tea daily (See Section Four).

3 - Drink three cups of couch-grass tea daily (See Section Four).

4 - Drink 25mls of celery juice, with the juice of one carrot and the juice from one handful of parsley.

5 - Combine two tablespoons of apple cider vinegar, one teaspoon of honey and one whole lemon juiced — add l00mls of water and drink daily.

Urinary tract - infection

◑ Caution

It is important to note that this is meant as a complementary formula and should be taken in conjunction with those medicines prescribed by your medical practitioner.

---

1 - Due to its medicinal actions, as a plant anti-biotic, the introduction of horseradish into your diet will assist with this condition. Horseradish can be eaten as a complementary addition to a main meal.

2 - Drink almond milk twice daily until condition is cleared (See Section Two).

3 - Drink couch-grass tea (See Section Four).

4 - Drink parsley tea (See Section Four).

5 - Introduce cauliflower into the diet.

6 - Drink 5mls of apple cider and 2.5mls of lemon juice with 20mls of water.

7 - Soak 1 tablespoon of black currants in 50mls of water and 5mls of apple cider vinegar. Leave

overnight and take each morning.

8 – Sip water throughout the day.

Urinary tract -inflammation

1 – Drink almond milk, with the combination of barley water (purchased from thesupermarket (See Section Two).

2 – When wanting to support any urinary tract problem or infection, introduce cauliflower into your diet. Combine this with dandelion leaf salad.

3 – Drink three cups of corn silk tea daily (See Section Four).

Urinary tract - maintaining a fluid balance

1 – Introduce cabbage regularly into your diet. This fluid balance assists the transportation of minerals in and out of cells.

Urinary tract - promoting the elimination of fluid

1 – Introduce globe artichoke into the diet.

2 – Introduce green beans into the diet.

3 – Introduce carrot regularly into the diet.

4 – The introduction of celery into your diet will help

eliminate the retention of fluid around the body.

5 - Introduce cucumber regularly into the diet.

6 - Introduce garlic and onion into your diet to help with the elimination of excessive fluid.

7 - Drink parsley tea (See Section Four).

8 - Drink apple peel tea daily (See Section Four).

9 - Introduce one eggplant into your daily diet to assist with urinary flow.

Urinary tract - spasm

1 - Drink almond milk (See Section Two).

2 - Drink corn silk tea (See Section Four).

Urinary tract - urinary sugar

1 - Introduce four or five asparagus stalks into your daily diet.

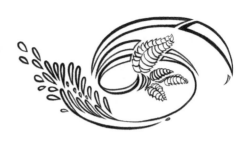

VAGINAL THRUSH

1 - Douche (purchase from chemist or use a sauce bottle and place contents in bottle or douche and flush morning and night) made with 200mls of water and 50mls of apple cider vinegar and 1 drop (only 1 drop) of eucalyptus oil. Apply daily

2 - Juice 1 leafy green and 1 stick of celery and take daily.

3 - Stop eating processed sugar and foods containing yeast.

4 - Reduce fruit.

5 - Reduce alcohol.

6 - Eat natural (non-flavoured yoghurt) daily.

7 - Wear cotton underwear avoiding nylon.

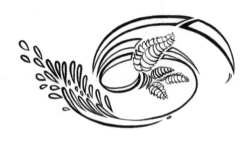

VITAMIN C DEFICIENCY

1 - Introduce celery into your diet.

2 - Introduce either whole or juiced apples, including the peel, into your daily diet.

3 - Eat plenty of fresh fruits and vegetables.

4 - Eat three kiwi fruit daily.

5 - Read up on foods listed in Section Two and smoothies and juices in Section Six.

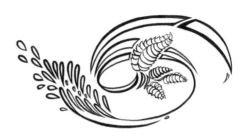

WARTS

1 – Tape banana peel to the wart with the white side against the skin and change the peel daily, after bathing.

2 – Introduce immune smoothies and juices to the diet (See Section Six).

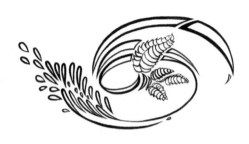

WORMS - INTESTINAL PARASITES

1 - Introduce carrot into the diet may help to control intestinal parasites or worms.

2 - Introduce dandelion leaves and calendula flowers regularly, as part of a fresh, leafy green salad.

3 - Introduce garlic into the diet may help to control this condition.

4 - Introduce pumpkin seeds to the diet.

5 - Juice ¼ onion and ¼ beetroot and 2 apples. Take on alternate days.

6 - Drink thyme tea (See Section Four).

WOUNDS - PARTICULARLY THOSE DIFFICULT OR SLOW TO HEAL

1 - Apply a poultice of pulped apple to the affected area, for several hours.

2 - Apply a paste of 2/3 apple and 1/3 garlic, with a small amount of olive oil, so as to avoid burning of the skin. Cover with gauze and leave for several hours.

3 - Apply mashed avocado to slow healing wounds, overnight.

4 - Apply a poultice of blackberry puree daily, to create a healing environment.

5 - Apply a cabbage poultice to the affected area.

6 - Squeeze lemon juice over the wound as a cleanser.

7 - Apply lavender oil to the affected area (See Section Five).

8 - Introduce sprouts and vegetable juices into the diet to activate internal healing.

*wounds must be closely monitored by your wholistically trained or medical practitioner.

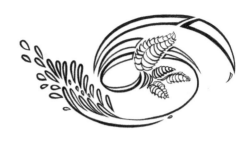

Section Two
Fruit And Vegetables

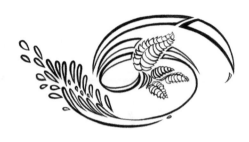

FRUIT AND VEGETABLES

It should be noted that this text focuses on the major constituents found within each fruit and vegetable and not every constituent is listed.

ALFALFA SPROUTS - *Medicago sativa*

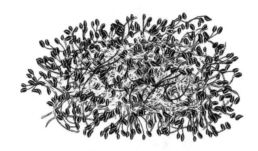

Alfalfa sprouts contain many health building properties and are helpful healing agents for many conditions.

Alfalfa aids cleansing and detoxifying of the body.

Alfalfa also introduces minerals into the body that are extremely important to general health.

Alfalfa has been found to contain some of the trace minerals, making it a totally nutritional food.

Mineral content: Calcium

Phosphorus

Iron

Potassium

Vitamin content: Vitamin A

Vitamin K

Vitamin D

ALMONDS -*Prunus amygdalus.*

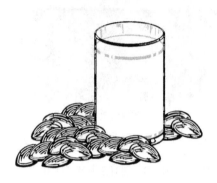

Almonds are a nutritionally balanced food.

Promote maximum absorption of the mineral matrix.

Contain a high level of oxalic acid, the blood clotting factor.

Contain 20% protein and consequently have been acknowledged by nutritionists as a good replacement for meat.

Mineral content:	Vitamin content:
Calcium	Vitamin A
Phosphorous	B Complex

Sulphur	Vitamin C -
Magnesium	almonds promote
Zinc	maximum absorption
Iron (a very small amount)	of Vitamin C
Chromium	
Acids:	Oxalic

Almond Milk Recipe

Ingredients: 50gms. raw almonds

50gms. honey (do not give to a baby under 12 months old, as they may demonstrate an allergic reaction) 1 litre water (for blending) extra water for soaking

Method: Place the raw almonds in water and leave for several hours.

Crush the almonds and blend in one litre of water. Filter the formula and stir in 1 tablespoon of honey, adding a little extra water. Allow formula to sit for several hours and strain.

Almond Puree

Ingredients: 10 almonds

A small amount of water.

Method: Place the almonds and the water in a blender and puree adding water as desired. Keep processing until a fine consistency is achieved.

APPLES–*Malus communis*

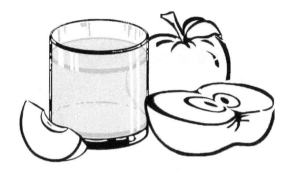

All apples contain the same properties. It is really a matter of personal preference and availability.

The apple contains a broad matrix of vitamins, minerals and nutrients.

Apple: *is a total health tonic

    *is safe for diabetics

    *is an astringent and therefore tightens tissues

    *stimulates the muscles and nerves into healing

    *will promote the elimination of fluid from the body

    *juice will eliminate uric acid from the blood

    *will cleanse the blood

*assists the body to balance and adapt

*The skin of the apple should not be peeled when juicing because the pectin is housed just under the skin layer.

Often the same benefits can be gained from eating the apple as from juicing it but you cannot consume the same amount.

Apples are regarded as one of the better anti-infective fruits.

Mineral content:	*Vitamin content:*
Iron	B Complex
Calcium	Vitamin A
Phosphorus	Vitamin C
Potassium	almonds promote
Magnesium	Vitamin G
	Vitamin B5
Acids:	Malic
Tartaric	Oxalic
Other nutrients:	Pectin
	Amino acids

APRICOTS *-Armenliaca vulgaris*

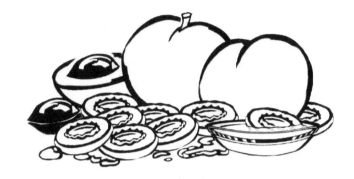

Apricots: *are a very nutritious food when fully ripened

*are easy to digest when fully ripened

*are very good for children, particularly those whose growth is retarded

*have been known to combat anaemia due to them containing a product called cobalt

*will develop healthy muscles and nerves

*will help to stimulate the appetite

*have been used favourably to treat bowel disorders

Fresh apricots are the primary choice. Dried apricots have six times the sugar content of fresh apricots.

Ten dried apricot halves will give you half the recommended daily quota of carotene.

Ten dried apricot halves will provide potassium and 20% of the recommended Iron allowance for men and post menopausal woman.

Mineral content: Potassium (Particularly in dried apricots.)

Iron Copper (Moderate source)

Cobalt

Calcium

Vitamin content: Vitamin B12 (Cobalt)

Vitamin A (Carotene)

Vitamin C

Amino acids

Reconstituting Dried Apricots

Dried fruit should be put in cold water and brought to the boil the night before, as the boiling kills any germs that may be on the fruit, or just soak over night, in water, before eating. Discard the water.

ASPARAGUS *-Asparagus officinalis*

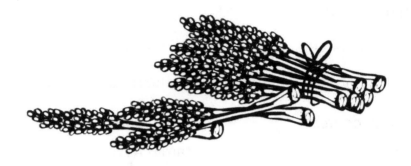

The healing powers of asparagus are nothing short of excellent.

Asparagus: *is a stimulant promotes normal bowel function

*assists to address constipation, diarrhoea ·and bowel diseases

*enhances liver function

*supports the heart and the arteries and assists to lower high cholesterol

*enhances the action of the kidney and the entire urinary tract

*should never be used in gout conditions due to the Purine it contains

It should be noted that taking too much asparagus can irritate the urinary tract, particularly if there is inflammation of the kidneys.

This vegetable assists in aiding the circulatory system. Avoid asparagus where there is acute rheumatism.

Mineral content:	*Vitamin content:*
Iron	Vitamin A
Chlorophyll	B Complex
Manganese	Vitamin C
Phosphorus	
Zinc	
Calcium	
Magnesium	
Manganese	

Acids

Uric Acid -   This is present as a result of a set of chemical compounds, called Purine, that converts into uric acid when in the system

Folic acid -

Other nutrients: Asparagine

Amino acids

AVOCADO *–Persea gratissima*

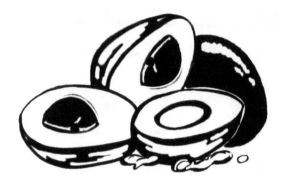

There are over four hundred varieties of avocado through-out the world. They all have different skins, texture of fruit, appearance and in some instances they even have a different flavour. All avocados are known as a neutral fruit. This means that they have a neutral flavour and can be used as a substitute for butter or margarine when used as a spread. It will blend with almost any flavour, whether sweet or savoury.

Avocado: *is regarded as a complete food and is very easily digested

*is very high in the amino acids that are essen-
tial to our body's function

*contains fats and these are classified as fruit
oils

*has a very high alkaline action

The seed offers healing.

Unlike most fruits, avocado contains very little sugar.

Avocado assists in addressing infections due to Colon Vacilli and Candida (Thrush), because of the unique anti-bacterial and anti-fungal substance that is found in the pulp.

This fruit is best eaten raw as the heating of it destroys the complex minerals. The structure of the fruit oil, found within the avocado, is also destroyed when heated.

Mineral content:

Avocado is very rich in mineral content.

Iron

Copper

Sodium and

Potassium

Vitamin content:

Vitamin C

Vitamin E

Vitamin B Complex

Vitamin A

Acids:

Amino	Folic Acid
in balance, which gives	
this food its very high	
Other nutrients:	Nerve Salts
alkaline action.	Fruit Oil
Magnesium	
Zinc	
Calcium	

BANANA -*Muser sapientum*

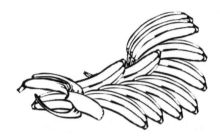

Bananas: *are a totally nutritional food, particularly when ripe

*are very rich in fibre and are easily digested

*are unsuitable for diabetics in large amounts

*are considered one of the better anti-infective fruits

*are often craved for in cases of thrush, or some other highly infected state

*are an instant energy boost, due to their high sugar content

*must be ripened naturally for easy digestion

*should be soft to the touch when right for eating

*feed the friendly intestinal flora

*assist the immune system due to their Vitamin C content

Some conditions react better to over ripe bananas because of the fibre changes the riper the banana gets, and the softer the plant the more it will absorb moisture to it.

Due to the carotene, which transfers to Vitamin A, this fruit is good as an anti— infective.

The Vitamin B Complexes are excellent for providing energy.

The sugars in the banana are readily assimilated.

When people are experiencing muscular problems bananas are also craved for, due to their high level of potassium.

Mineral content: Calcium (approx. twenty four milli-grams per five hundred gms)

Phosphorus (approx. eighty five milli-grams per five hundred gms)

Potassium

	Magnesium
	Manganese
	Selenium
	Zinc (low)
Vitamin content:	Vitamin A (Carotene)
	B Complex
	Vitamin C
Acids:	Folic acid
	Amino acids

BARLEY –*Hordeum vulgare*

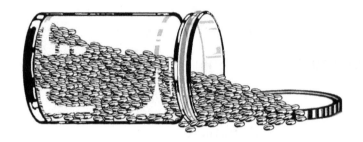

Barley is highly regarded as effective to treat a broad range of conditions. The general use of barley is to address aggravated conditions, in particular stomach ulcers, diarrhoea, gallstones and bronchial spasms. Barley reduces bile acid secretion and may assist in lowering LDL (the bad guy) in the cholesterol chain.

Barley water is also an effective preparation in convalescence and is an effective alkaliser.

Mineral content: Calcium

Iron

Phosphorus

Manganese

Selenium

Magnesium

Potassium

Vitamin content: Thiamine

Riboflavin

Niacin

B6

Other: Insoluble fibre

Folic acid

BEANS -*Phaseolus vulgaris*

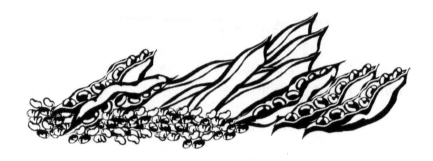

Beans: *stimulate normal nerve function

*promote the elimination of excess fluids

*are one of the most powerful medicines for the entire cardiovascular system

*aid normal bowel function due to their fibrous content

*help to detoxify the body

*on a regular, preferably daily basis, will assist in building the blood

Beans can often cause people to have gas. It has been suggested, by researchers in the United States, that proper soaking of the bean will rid it of most of its gas producing potential. Frequent eating of beans will increase the enzyme function.

Of the body and therefore the body will develop a tolerance. In most conditions treated with beans, the beans are
either raw or juiced.

The bean will assist the function and regeneration of
the liver.

Due to their assistance in the general function of the
liver, the bean will help with the residual side effects of
cortisone.

A cup of beans daily will help to regulate the insulin
through the pancreas.

Bean juice can be combined with carrot, apple and celery juices.

Mineral content:	The string of the bean has the highest mineral content of the whole plant.
Vitamin content:	Vitamin A
	B Complex
	Vitamin C - potent
Other nutrients	Pectin
	Gum
	Chlorophyll-in the actual bean

BEETROOT - *Beta ruba*

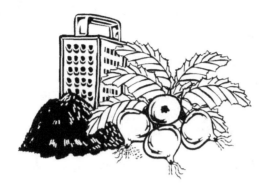

Beetroot:*is very easily digested is a blood builder and a blood tonic

   *is regarded as a blood cleanser, liver tonic and kidney support

   *is very nutritious and regarded by nutritionists, as one of the best appetite stimulants

   *contains lime, which helps to break down pathogenic waste

   *regenerates healthy liver cells

   *should be used in all hepatitis conditions

The magnesium in beetroot assists in the treatment of depression and anxiety. Some research has favourably reported the value of beetroot in assisting with, or the prevention of, cancers and leukemic states.

Diabetics should only consume small amounts of beetroot juice, because of the high sugar content.

Tinned beetroot is usually in vinegar and the vinegar decreases oxygen uptake and it can make you sluggish. Beetroot is best if you prepare it yourself by gently roasting, steaming, eating raw or juicing.

Mineral content: Magnesium

Manganese

Sodium

Potassium

Phosphorus

Iron

Vitamin content: Vitamin A - very high

Vitamin C

Vitamin B Complex

Other nutrients: Alkaloid Betaine

BLACKBERRIES *–Rubus fructicosus*

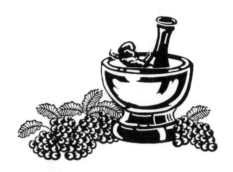

Blackberries: *are regarded as a noxious weed but they are in fact quite a powerful medicine

*are regarded as one of the better anti-infective fruits

*are a highly nutritious food

*contains isocitric acid

*also contains glycosides which are active constituents that give the blackberry a broad range of action

*contain natural sugars

*contain pectin

* assist the body to utilise iron.

Blackberry is classified as an astringent which has the ability to heal wounds by drawing tissues together.

Mineral content:	Vitamin content:
Salts	Vitamin A
Iron	Natural Oils
	Vitamin C
	Vitamin E
Other nutrients:	Glycosides
	Gum
	Natural Sugars
	Pectin
Acids:	Malic

Blackberry Root Powder

Dig up the root and thinly slice it. Leave it outside in the sun on a mesh tray and when it has dried, powder down using a pestle and mortar.

Dried Blackberry Formula

Find a blackberry bush, that you know has not been sprayed. Dry the berries, the leaves and the root and then powder. When suffering from diarrhoea, sore throat or sinus, you can take it by the teaspoon or in a small amount of water.

Alternatively, sprinkle on food.

Drying the formula does not alter the mineral matrix.

BROCCOLI -*Brassica oleracea italica*

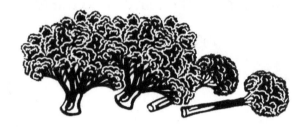

It is the sulphur content in broccoli that provides the healing potential.

Broccoli is known to activate gas producing enzymes and this creates a problem for some people. To help avoid this when cooking the broccoli, steam it with a piece of parchment paper lining the steamer and put the broccoli on top of the paper. The parchment paper will absorb the agent that produces the gas. The other alternative is to eat it raw, or soak for several hours before steaming. Slow cooking reduces the possibility of producing gas.

Broccoli: *is of benefit for muscular development

*beneficial for the glands of the body, especially those that aid in the digestion of food

Within the family of broccoli we have:

- Cabbage
- Brussel sprouts
- Cauliflower

The high levels of chlorophyll finds broccoli to be an extremely effective cancer blocking formula. If you have a genetic link to cancer, drinking of a juice that contains broccoli, cabbage, beans, carrot and apple provides a line of defence for the fighting of mutant cells. Russian literature supports the research that broccoli is an effective treatment for Cervical Cancer. This study goes back to 1952, and has been reported many times since in both science and medical magazines and journals.(Heinerman reports on Federation Proceedings (May 1976), Cancer Research (May 1978), Science News(April 13, 1985).

For those conditions that can be assisted with the introduction of broccoli into the diet, broccoli should be eaten three times a week.

Mineral content:

Sulphur

Potassium

Phosphorus

Calcium

Iron

Other nutrients:

Vitamin content:

Vitamin A
(3,500international

Units per 5000gms.)

Vitamin B (Thlamlne)

Vitamin C

Vitamin E

Vitamin K

Chlorophyll

CABBAGE -*Brassica oleracea*

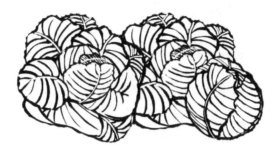

Cabbage: *very similar to broccoli, so too is brussel sprouts

*is regarded as an eye strengthener

*is excellent to treat iron deficiency

*has excellent healing properties

*has an anti-inflammatory action

*can be used to treat a broad range of conditions

*assists in the elimination of waste throughout the body

Due to its drawing strength, cabbage has the ability to draw pathogenic waste. The therapeutic use of cabbage is so extensive that books have been written on its healing properties and uses.

It is the combination of chlorine, potassium and sodium found in the cabbage that makes it such a good digestive aid, blended with chlorophyll.

Because of its high mineral content cabbage is particularly good for healthy hair, teeth and nails.

Mineral content:	*Vitamin content:*
Chlorine	Vitamin C
Potassium	Vitamin B1
Sodium	Vitamin B2
Iron	Vitamin B3
Calcium	Vitamin A
Phosphorus	Vitamin U
	Vitamin K
Acids:	Hydrochloric
Other nutrients:	Chlorophyll

CALENDULA FLOWERS *–Calendula officinalis*

Calendula flowers are a useful antiseptic and first-aid remedy.

The Vitamins C and A that are found in the flower enables this part of the plant to act as a cleanser and together with the phosphorus, also assists the immune system.

The flower head provides an antiseptic oil that has extraordinary healing abilities.

Mineral content: Phosphorus

Vitamin content: Vitamin A

                    Vitamin C

Other nutrients: fixed oil

CANTALOUPE *Cucumis melo*

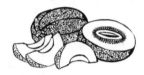

Cantaloupe is noted by natural medicine consultants around the globe to be an exceptional fruit to aid healing. This is due to the impressive nutrients that are housed within the product. Eaten fresh on a regular basis and partnered with cherries, pineapple, avocado and mint leaves proves to support the body, in particular the digestive system.

Mineral content: Phosphorus

Calcium

Iron

Potassium

Vitamin content: Vitamin A

Vitamin C

Vitamin B group

CARROT-*Daucus carota*

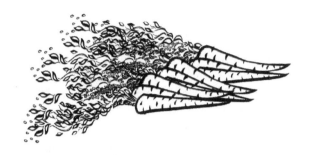

There are many different varieties of carrot and the one you choose to eat should be governed purely by taste preference and availability.

Carrot contains a very high amount of beta-carotene, converting to Vitamin A as it passes through the body.

Excessive consumption of carrots should be avoided as the body may have difficulty assimilating the beta-carotene.

Carrot has an alkaloid that may turn the skin yellow. This chemical is called Daucarine and it is poisonous in large amounts. It does however, assist the circulatory system. Research has found it to be a vasodilator.

In sensible doses the carrot assists the health of the arteries.

Carrot: *is an anti-oxidant and general cleanser

        *is excellent for healthy skin and hair

        *is an excellent source of minerals

        *provides energy

        *regulates intestinal activity

        *is an excellent anti-inflammatory

        *the seeds are overlooked for their extraordinary drawing power

The pancreas, gall bladder and liver are all organs that will respond well to the introduction of carrot into your diet.

Mineral content: Iron

                Phosphorus

                Calcium

                Sodium

                Potassium

                Magnesium

                Arsenic (a trace process by attaching element)

                Manganese

                Sulphur

Vitamin content: Vitamin A - Carotene
                     Vitamin B Complex
                     Vitamin C

Other nutrients: Asparagine - facilitates healing
                     Daucasine - an alkaloid which provides
                     an anti-inflammatory action

CAULIFLOWER -*Brassica oleracea*

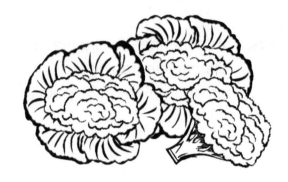

Cauliflower's key function is to support the urinary tract

Cauliflower is in the cabbage family.

The molecular structure of the cauliflower is very similar to that of the cabbage. Cauliflower is best eaten raw for the vitamin and mineral content.

Cauliflower introduces a good amount of fibre into the diet.

When steaming cauliflower always put the green leaf with it because the minerals are housed within the green leaves that are on the outside of the vegetable.

If there are not enough green leaves on the outside then use cabbage leaves.

Due to the high sulphur content in cauliflower it can be difficult to assimilate so you should have small, raw pieces.

Mineral content: Potassium (very high)
Iron
Sulphur
Calcium
Phosphorous
Zinc

Vitamin content: Vitamin A
Vitamin B1
Vitamin B2
Vitamin B3
Vitamin C

CAYENNE *–Capsicum annum*

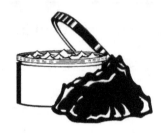

Cayenne powder is a natural stimulant, heating the body, and helping it overcome flu and colds. Cayenne also assists the digestive process and aids in the reduction of flatulence.

Mineral content:	Iron
	Calcium
	Sulphur
	Magnesium
	Potassium
Vitamin content:	Vitamin A
	Vitamin C
	Vitamin B Complex

Cayenne Lotion

Ingredients: Cayenne powder

Sorbalene

Method: Mix one part Cayenne powder to ten parts of

Sorbalene.

CELERY –*Apium graveolens*

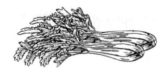

Celery: *is used as a complementary addition to many formulas

    *is a general cleanser of the body

    *is a high alkaline forming food

When using celery to assist with any condition you should use both the leaf and the stalk.

When using celery for therapeutic uses it should never be cooked. It is high in calcium and as calcium is lost under heat, consuming celery in a raw or juiced state is preferred.

Celery acts as an anti-inflammatory.

Mineral content: Iron

    Calcium

    Magnesium

    Sodium

    Phosphorous

Vitamin content: Vitamin A

Vitamin B Complex

Vitamin C

CHERRIES -*Cerasus vulgaris*

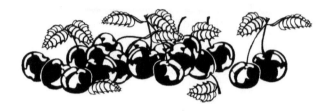

Cherries are favourably reported in folk medicine texts.

Cherries have been prescribed throughout many cultures for conditions where there is nutritional insufficiency, but recently has been found that cherries contains bio-flavonoids. These are nutritional agents that assist the body to recover from illness.

The healing ability of cherries is attributed to the complex chemistry of this fruit that enables it to act as an anti-inflammatory agent.

Vitamin P has been isolated in cherries and this Vitamin has been found to be of benefit to the arteries, veins and the capillaries. The introduction of cherries into the diet for inflammatory conditions, such as gout, arthritis or convalescence, has shown to produce significant results.

Mineral content:	Iron
	Copper
	Manganese
Vitamin content:	Vitamin A
	Vitamin C
Other nutrients:	Bio-flavonoids

CHILLI – *Capsicum annum*

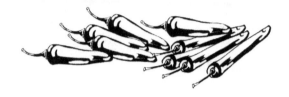

    Chilli is assessed for its heat and rated on a scale called the Scoville Units. Mild to moderate, hot and very hot is the range. Therapeutically chilli is a powerful healer. Be careful handling chilli and start on the lower heat chillies to gauge your tolerance. A little goes a long why. Include in cooking, juices and smoothies to aid circulation and clearing of congestion in the body. The red chilli is usually higher in nutrients. If the mouth burns from too much chilli have a glass of full cream milk or 50gms of plain yoghurt.

Mineral content: Iron

                        Copper

                        Potassium

Vitamin content: Vitamin C (high)

Vitamin A

Vitamin B group

Other nutrients: Bio-flavonoids

Capsaicin

CLOVES -*Sygizium aromaticum*

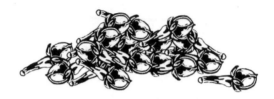

A wonderful pain reliever and decongestant clove offers exceptional healing. Where the body is generally debilitated and struggling to recuperate the wonderful little clove bud can activate the healing process.

The literature suggests the powerful healing is confirmed as the active principles are known to provide healing properties such as antioxidant, local anaesthetic, antiseptic+ anti-inflammatory and carminative and digestive settling properties. In addition to the internal response to the consumption of cloves, topically they produce a rubefacient response (warming),

Mineral content: Magnesium

Potassium

Iron

	Selenium
	Manganese
Vitamin content:	A
	C
	B1 and B6
	K
Other:	Essential oils
	Flavonoids
	Triterpenes

CORN -*Zea mays*

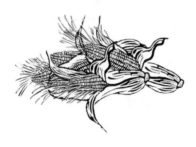

Corn silk is commonly used in clinical practice pre-scribed as a tea to assist recovery from conditions affecting the urinary system.

Corn: *is a nutritious vegetable due to its complex range of vitamins and minerals

*is a general tonic and a body building food

Corn must be chewed thoroughly to ensure assimila-tion.

This vegetable is best eaten raw, or lightly steamed, because the thiamine content is reduced dramatically by cooking.

Mineral content:	Iron
	Calcium
	Phosphorus
Vitamin content:	Vitamin B Complex
	Vitamin A
	Niacin
	Thiamine (B1)
Other nutrients:	Complex formulation of Natural Sugars.
	Mineral salts.

CUCUMBER –*Cucumis melo*

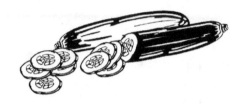

Cucumber would be one of the most popular diuretics (reducing fluid).

The potassium content of this vegetable makes it suitable for treating both high and low blood pressure.

Cucumber contains a particular enzyme that breaks down protein.

The high mineral content of cucumber makes it an excellent vegetable for the elimination of uric acid.

Mineral content: Potassium

Silicon

Sulphur

Phosphorus

Calcium

Manganese

Vitamin content: Vitamin A

Vitamin B Complex

Vitamin C

Other nutrients: Erepsin - assists in breaking down protein.

CURRANTS – *Ribes nigrum*

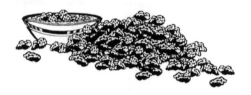

There is often confusion between raisins, sultanas and currants. Raisins are dried white grapes, sultanas are dried seedless grapes and currants are dried dark red seedless grapes. All are very nutritious and healing and may be used in combination with each other.

Currants have been recognised by many cultures to have wonderful healing properties, in particular antiseptic properties. In addition the nutritional elements are without question why these little gems are so magnificent as a healing remedy.

Research confirms that it is the GLA (gamma linolenic acid) content that is responsible for such positive healing responses.

Mineral content:	Calcium
	Iron
	Phosphorus
Vitamin content:	A
	B group
	C
Other:	See Section Four for an old arthritic remedy Gin-Soaked Raisin Remedy

DANDELION *-Taraxacum officinalis*

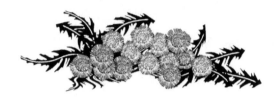

This is perhaps one of the most balanced nutritional substances in the plant kingdom, particularly when using the whole plant, including both the root and the leaves. The root can be steamed like parsnip, and the leaves can be used in salads, as a bitter digestive aid used to accompany meals and assisting in the digestive process when eating meat.

As a general cleanser of the system it is unsurpassed.

Mineral content: Iron

Magnesium

Potassium

Sodium

Silica

Zinc

Calcium

Vitamin content: Vitamin A

Vitamin C

Vitamin B Complex

Vitamin E

Other nutrients: Chlorophyll

Dandelion Drink Recipe

Ingredient: The whole fresh root and leaves.

Method: Wash the whole plant and then juice.

DATES -*Phoenix dactylifera*

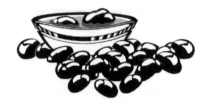

Dates are a very easy to digest food, very nutritious and a food to aid convalescence. All parts of the body respond well to the introduction of dates into the diet, in particular the bowel.

Mineral content: Iron

Magnesium

Phosphorous

Potassium

Calcium

Vitamin content: Vitamin A

Vitamin C

Vitamin B Complex

Other nutrients: Amino acids

EGGPLANT -*Solanum melongena*

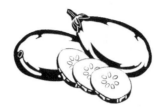

Eggplant: *is in the potato family.

     *to be baked as it is easier to digest

     *will assist the liver and the pancreas to perform
      to their optimum

One of the natural benefits is that it combats anaemia

Mineral content: Iron

                   Phosphorous

                   Calcium

                   Potassium

Vitamin content: Vitamin A

                   Vitamin B1

                   Vitamin B2

                   Vitamin B3

                   Vitamin C

Other nutrients: Polyphenols; Anthocyanins and chloro-

genic acid are effective antioxidants and

anti-inflammatory compounds

FENNEL *Foeniculum vulgare*

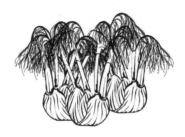

Fennel is gaining popularity as the Australian palate expands. It is truly a remarkable plant and one where every part can be used. The seeds offer a powerful action to settle the digestive system while the stalk and leaves act as gentle support to the digestive process.

The diversity of fennel is supported by the fact it offers healing to the entire body acting as a healing and health providing food specifically directed to the immune, digestive, cardio-vascular and musculo-skeletal systems.

Mineral content: Zinc

Phosphorous

Selenium

Potassium

	Iron
	Sodium
	Calcium
	Magnesium
Vitamin content:	Beta-carotene
	C
	E
	K
	B3
	B5
Other nutrients:	Natural source of plant estrogen
	Aromatic oils such as anethole
	Amino acids (histidine, arginine)

FIGS –*Ficus carica*

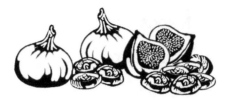

Figs are a nutritional food.

When fresh figs are in season most nutritionalists would recommend they should be eaten regularly, particularly by growing children, due to their high mineral content. Figs are easily eaten by children because they are sweet.

Figs that are sun dried will not lose their nutritional value.

Figs contain a nutritional element called ficins, which helps the digestive process. The enzymes in figs enable them to be very effective in the treatment of constipation.

Figs contain valuable alkaline product and will be of benefit in the treatment of acidic conditions.

Mineral content:	Iron
	Calcium
	Manganese
	Potassium
	Copper
	Sodium
Vitamin content:	Vitamin A
	Vitamin B Complex (High in B1, B2, B6)
	Vitamin C
Other nutrients:	A mix of enzymes.
	Ficins

GARLIC -*Allium sativum* & ONION-*Allium cepa*

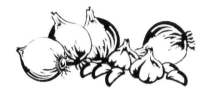

Garlic and onion can be linked together as they have similar properties. If you look at their botanical names you will see they are from the same family. Due to the broad range of medicinal uses the garlic and the onion plays a significant role in natural medicine. Research has been indicating the onion may be even better than the garlic.

◑ **Note**

It is important to note that one major difference when using garlic for external poultice combinations is to not apply it direct to the skin. First you must smear the area with oil as the sulphur in the garlic is very powerful and may burn the skin.

Onion on the other hand, has a smoother and a softer oil, and is not as harsh as the garlic.

The odour that is given off by the garlic is caused by the meeting of two enzymes. Cutting a clove of garlic in half will activate the odorous enzymes. If you can avoid bruising the garlic you will reduce the odour. A European way of eating garlic is to take one whole clove, not bruised, wrap it in a piece of bread and swallow it like a tablet, this will greatly reduce the odour.

If you do activate the odorous enzymes, the eating of orange peel, parsley or mint, after the consumption of the garlic, will help to eliminate the odour fairly quickly. If you can smell garlic on yourself then the dose range is too high.

The volatile oil that is found within the garlic is excreted from the body via the lungs. The healing takes place as the product is excreted from the body, hence mouth odour.

One of the greatest enhances of the immune system is garlic

Garlic has been referred to as nature's penicillin

Garlic will assist the body to lower the production of excess mucous.

Garlic will assist the body to expectorate phlegm.

All types of infection, be they internal, external, local or wide spread, can be assisted with the use of garlic.

Onions are a wonderful cleanser due to antiseptic oils that are found naturally in this vegetable.

It has been well documented that these oils reduce blood clots in the body.

Heart patients should consider this food on a daily basis. Start with small amounts in a salad and increase as tolerance is gained.

It is preferable if onions are eaten raw, but also include them in cooking.

Mineral content:

Garlic	Onion
Selenium	Potassium
Iron	Phosphorus
Potassium	Iodine
Zinc	Nickel
Calcium	Silicon
Manganese	Zinc
Sulphur	Iron
Magnesium	

Vitamin content:

Garlic	Onion
Vitamin A	Vitamin E
Vitamin C	Vitamin A
Vitamin B1	Thiamine (B1)
Thiamine (B1)	Riboflavin
	Niacin
	Vitamin C

Onion and Garlic Soup Recipe.

Ingredients: 2 large onions

500mls. chicken stock

garlic

pepper

Method: Finely slice the onion and heat with garlic in a large pan. Add the chicken stock and pepper and allow to heat and simmer for five to ten minutes.

Onion Syrup Formula

Ingredients: Onions

Brown sugar

Method: Peel and thinly slice the onion and lay it on a tray . Sprinkle a light layer of brown sugar over the onion and allow it to sit for a few hours. When you return a syrup will have formed from the sugar filtering through the onion rings.

or

Method: Invert one bowl, inside a larger bowl. Using the onion rings layer them inside one bowl and sprinkle sugar in between each layer. The onion juice and sugar will filter through the layers and form a syrup in the bottom of the bowl.

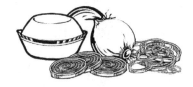

Onion and Honey Syrup Recipe

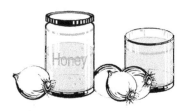

Ingredients: Onions and honey.

Method: Juice the onions and combine with honey, using two thirds of a cup of juice and one third of a cup of honey.

GINGER *Zingiber officinalis*

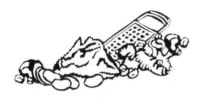

Ginger root is invaluable as a source of powerful healing products and is versatile in the many ways it can be used and utilised on a daily basis.

A warming product offering many body systems an opportunity to heal when ginger is ingested.

Mineral content: Zinc

Sodium

Calcium

Potassium

Magnesium

Phosphorous

Iron

Vitamin content:	B6
	C
	Niacin
	Folate
Other nutrients:	Phenolic compounds

GLOBE ARTICHOKE–*Cynara scolymus*

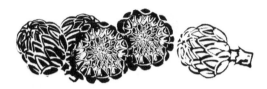

This vegetable assists in the treatment of and support to the liver.

Globe artichoke:

       *assists in the treatment of the gall bladder

       *is easily digested.

       *is an excellent source of energy.

If you have any conditions that can be assisted by eating globe artichoke then try to make it part of your daily diet.

Mineral content: Manganese

                         Phosphorus

                         Iron

                         Zinc

Vitamin content: Vitamin A

Vitamin B Complex

Vitamin C

Other nutrients: Inulin and Cinarin are carbohydrates and can be assimilated by diabetics as suggested by Jean Valnet with the highest content in the leaves.

GRAPEFRUIT -*Citrus decumana*

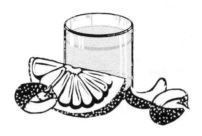

Due to the chemistry of grapefruit it is excellent for purification of the body.

Its high content of Vitamin A helps to support the immune system.

Most of the essential oils in this fruit are housed in the skin, and is necessary to incorporate the skin when juicing. These oils act as an antiseptic and a general body cleanser.

Mineral content: Calcium

Phosphorus

Potassium

Magnesium

	Iron
	Sodium
Vitamin content:	Vitamin A
	Vitamin C
	Biotin B5
Other nutrients:	Essential Oils
	Pectins

> Be cautious when taking some pharmaceuticals as they may conflict with grapefruit.
> Peel and remove the pith (the white part under the skin) as it is bitter.

HORSERADISH –*Armoracia rusticana*

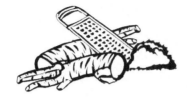

Horseradish: ∗has a powerful antibiotic action

∗acts as a general cleanser and clears the system of infection

∗is excellent for clearing the nasal passages and the sinuses generally

∗is a rich source of Vitamin C and B1

This vegetable has a significant benefit on the digestive system.

Mineral content: Sulphur

Potassium

Iron

Sodium

Calcium

Phosphorus

Vitamin content:	Vitamin A
	Vitamin B Complex
	Vitamin B1
	Vitamin C
	Vitamin P
Other nutrients:	Fixed oils

KALE–*Brassica oleracea var. sabellia*

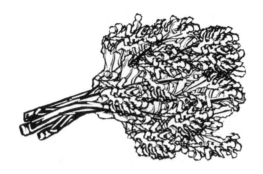

Kale is becoming much more popular as a leafy green to add to the diet as people realise the importance of including greens into their daily diet. Kale offers healing to the entire body as it helps the blood to rejuvenate. For all cases where the body requires healing the introduction of kale would be invaluable.

*Please note it is imperative you lightly steam kale prior to juicing, blending or eating in any form so as to avoid problems that may develop with thyroid function. (University of Queensland, Gatton campus research).

Mineral content:	Potassium
	Iron
	Calcium
Vitamin content:	Vitamin K
	Vitamin A
	Vitamin C
Other:	Omega − fatty acids 3 − 6
	Phenolic compounds
	Flavonoids in particular quercetin

KIWI FRUIT–*Actinidia chinensis*

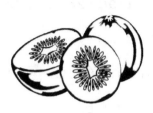

Kiwi fruit: ∗is very high in Vitamin C content

∗is very high in fibre

∗a wonderful digestive aid

Eating the whole fruit is excellent for the bowel to operate efficiently.

Due to its nutritional matrix this fruit is excellent for the skin, the immune, circulatory and digestive systems.

Adding kiwi fruit to your diet will assist in the management of emotional stress.

The high potassium levels in kiwi fruit are of benefit to increase energy levels. Excellent fibre content.

Mineral content: Potassium levels are high

(average 250mgs per kiwi fruit)

Sodium

Vitamin content: Vitamin C levels very high

Vitamin E

Other: Inositol is a sugar alcohol that naturally

occurs in kiwifruit

LEMON -*Citrus limonum*

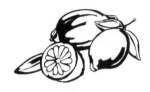

Lemon: *is excellent for gastro intestinal tract cleansing

*is a blood purifier, destroying harmful bacteria

*is a liver cleanser

*is metabolised by the body as alkaline

When juicing, include the rind. This acts as a cleanser and antiseptic.

Mineral content: Potassium

Calcium

Iron

Phosphorus

Vitamin content: Vitamin C

Vitamin B3 - Niacin

Thiamine (B1)

Riboflavin - refer to B2

Other nutrients: Bio-flavonoids - refer to Vitamin P

Lemon and Honey Syrup

Ingredients: The juice of three raw lemons, including peel, ½ cup of honey 1 litre of water

Method: Blend all the ingredients together. This may be consumed hot or cold. To dilute add ½ a cup of boiling water to ½ a cup of syrup.

Roasted lemons

Ingredients: 3 whole lemons unpeeled

Method: Place a fine cut into the peel of the lemons to allow for expansion as they cook. Place lemons on a small rack over water to allow cooking to be over steam. Roast the lemons until soft. Allow to cool. Place the lemons and the water from the dish into a blender and blend. Place in an airtight jar, refrigerate and use as needed. Honey may be added after cooling.

LETTUCE–*Lactuca sativa*

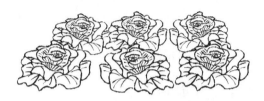

Lettuce has been used as a sedative and as a cough suppressant.

The outer green leaves of the lettuce are the most nutritious.

Lettuce is one of the best sources of Iron.

The fact that lettuce is rarely cooked renders it a very valuable, mineral rich food.

Mineral content: Iron

Magnesium

Calcium

Phosphorus

Potassium

Zinc

Iodine

Silicon

Sulphur

Vitamin content: Vitamin A

Vitamin C

Vitamin D

Vitamin E

Vitamin B Complex

Other nutrients: Chlorophyll

LOQUAT-*Eriobotrya japonica*

Loquat is a fruit that has been gathering scientific credibility, yet it is a prized medicine from many cultures and has stood the test of time as a powerful medicine. Although the entire plant is researched it is mainly the leaves and fruit that are used although the seeds have healing properties.

Loquats: *have been reported to assist in the treatment of:

*diarrhoea

*elevating moods

*fluid retention

*type 11 diabetes support to the pancreas

*pancreatin health

*liver health

*skin support for dry, red and inflamed

*immune health

Mineral content:	Calcium
	Iron
	Phosphorous
	Potassium
Vitamin content:	Vitamin A
	Vitamin C
Other:	Pectin

> Grow a loquat tree or find a neighbour who has one and share the leaves and fruit. Always scrape off the fine hairs from the leaf before use. Dry the leaf and use as a tea.

LYCEE *Litchi clunenses*

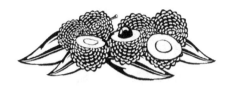

Fresh lychee is an excellent digestive aid and very palatable. Combines well with pawpaw, papaya, pineapple and or mint.

Mineral content: Iron

Phosphorous

Potassium

Copper

Vitamin content: Vitamin C

B group

Other nutrients: Oligonol, an antioxidant

MANGO *Mangifera indica*

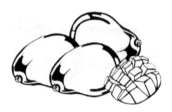

Mango has been used as a powerful medicine by many cultures throughout the ages. Generally mango offers valuable nutrients that aid the kidneys, the digestive system, and assist the bowel to perform to its optimum. The inner skin applied to dry, scaly, irritated skin may offer soothing relief.

Mineral content: Iron

Phosphorous

Calcium

Potassium

Copper

Vitamin content: Vitamin C

Vitamin A

Vitamin B group

Other nutrients: Antioxidants such as zeaxanthin

OLIVE–*Olea europaea*

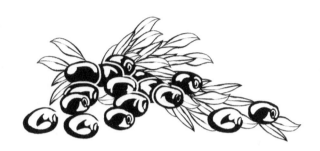

The olive tree is truly a medicine cabinet all rolled into one magnificent tree. The fruit, leaves and the bark are called upon in herbal medicine. Topically the oil is excellent for the skin and internally the oil aids the digestive process especially the function of the gallbladder, the liver and the heart.

The leaves are used by herbalists to make tinctures and infusions, providing a valuable treatment to support the immune system

Mineral content: Sodium

Potassium

Calcium

Iron

Magnesium

Phosphorous

Vitamin content: Vitamin A

Vitamin B6 and B12

Vitamin C

Vitamin D

Other nutrients: Antioxidants such as oleuropein and oleocanthal acting also as an anti-inflammatory.

ORANGE -*Citrus auranrium*

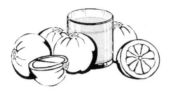

Oranges have been reported to:

> *assist in the reduction of cholesterol

> *reduce catarrh

> *assist in improving the immune system

Oranges will assist the reduction of excessive mucous following the common cold or influenza.

Orange peel has the remarkable ability to reduce indigestion.

Orange eaten in segments, not juiced, is good for constipation.

Orange peel acts as an anti-histamine.

Mineral content: Calcium

Iron

Phosphorous

	Potassium
	Sodium
Vitamin content:	Vitamin A
	Vitamin B1, B2, B3
	Vitamin C
Other nutrients:	Fruit Oils

PARSLEY–*Apium petroselinum*

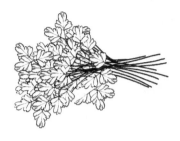

There are many types of parsley.

It is very high in both Vitamin C and A and this makes it a powerful immune stimulant and anti-oxidant herb.

Parsley's high content of chlorophyll is why it is a good blood builder and cleanser. The plant estrogens that are contained in parsley assist the female reproductive system.

Mineral content: Iodine

Manganese

Potassium

Calcium

Iron

	Phosphorus
	Magnesium
Vitamin content:	Vitamin A
	Vitamin B Complex
	Vitamin C
Other Nutrients:	Enzymes
	Essential Oils
	Plant Estrogens
	Chlorophyll

PAWPAW -*Carica papaya*

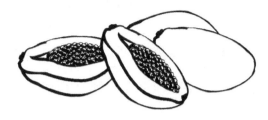

This food must be eaten when soft as the healing components are not active, nor the enzymes complete, when not fully ripened.

Papain is a digestive aid found in this fruit. Papain has the ability to tenderise hard to digest foods.

Pawpaw has been found to break down meat particles if the meat is marinated in pawpaw cubes before cooking. This makes the meat easier to digest. Papain is the powerful enzyme that produces the significant response by the digestive system. Fibrin, a rare chemical component that can be found in some plants, is in pawpaw. It affects the blood clotting process.

Pawpaw also contains Arginine, which is a chemical component that is exceptional for male fertility.

Another enzyme called Carpaine is thought to be helpful for the heart. (The Book of Raw Fruit and Vegetable Juices and Drink, by William H. Lee.)

Mineral content: Sodium

Calcium

Phosphorus

Potassium

Iron

Magnesium

Vitamin content: Vitamin A

Vitamin C

Acids: **Amino Acid**

Arginine

Carpaine

Fibrin

PEAR *Pyrus commmunis*

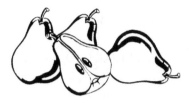

This pleasant tasting fruit must be eaten ripe where the full healing benefits can be achieved. You know when it is ripe enough when you can eat it off a spoon, good juice flows.

The digestive system performs well in the pathway of pears and the bowel can balance very well when pears are included in the daily diet. Reports of soothing colitis by eating ripe pears is common while assisting the break down of mucosal congestion.

Mineral content: Iron

Calcium

Phosphorous

Potassium

Vitamin content: Vitamin C

Vitamin A

Vitamin B

Other nutrients: Flavonoids to aid type 11 diabetes

Anti-inflammatory

Antioxidant

PEPPERMINT *LEAVES–Mentha piperita*

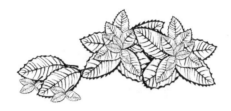

Peppermint leaves have been found to strengthen and cleanse the entire body. Peppermint leaves are calming to the stomach and are of assistance to bowel function. They are a powerful digestive aid.

Mineral content: Iron

Sulphur

Silicon

Potassium

Niacin

Iodine

Magnesium

Vitamin content: Vitamin C

Vitamin A

Other nutrients: Complex Oils

Menthol

PINEAPPLE–*Ananas sativus*

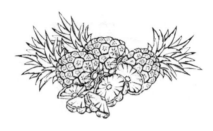

Pineapple must be eaten fresh if maximum nutritional value is to be gained from the introduction of this fruit into your diet.

Pineapple contains a powerful digestive aid, called Bromelain. The combination of both pineapple and paw-paw juice creates a dynamic healer and digestive agent.

Pineapple, when fresh, has a very high content of Vitamin C. This Vitamin C content assists the plant to be used in the management and discomfort of a sore throat. Pineapple will help to break down mucous acting as an expectorant.

Pineapple is used-as a diuretic, (the release of fluid).

The significant vitamin content of the pineapple provides the ability to enhance the function of the immune system.

Mineral content: Sulphur

Iron

Calcium

Phosphorus

Potassium

Manganese

Magnesium

Iodine

Vitamin content: Vitamin A

Vitamin B Complex

Vitamin C

Other nutrients: The enzyme Bromelain.

POMEGRANATE–*Punica granatum*

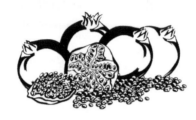

Pomegranate is a great tasting and medicinal plant. The fruit is packed with nutrients and healing agents. Research supports the use of pomegranate juice to support the heart and blood vessels.

Mineral content: Magnesium

Iron

Calcium

Sodium

Potassium

Vitamin content: Vitamin B6 and B - 12

Vitamin C

Vitamin D

Vitamin A

Other nutrients: Punicalagin

POTATO -*Solanum tuberosum*

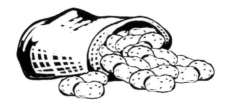

Potato is a very complex food. It contains a blend of chemistry that supports Its use as a powerful healing substance.

Potatoes have been found to be high in vitamins, mineral salts and carbohydrates

This makes the potato a nutritious food.

Some people can be allergic to potato if they have an allergy to sulphur based foods.

History confirms the nutritious benefit of potato as cultures have survived simply by having potato as their staple diet.

Mineral content: Sodium

Calcium

Magnesium

Copper

Sulphur

Manganese

Iron

Vitamin content: Vitamin B Complex

Vitamin C

Vitamin D

Vitamin A

PRUNES–*Prunus domestica*

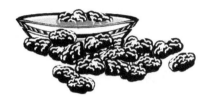

Prunes offer a wealth of healing, however many people avoid them due to the fact they usually take in too many. Prunes are the dried fruit of the plum and valued the world over by natural medicine practitioners.

As the blood is the river of life prunes offer outstanding benefits in providing a tonic to the blood stream where wellbeing and vitality can be achieved.

The most common use of prunes is to treat stubborn constipation. It is imperative that the 'less is more' approach is adopted.

◑ Use

Soak 3 prunes in 150mls of cold water and leave overnight. Add 1 teaspoon of apple cider vinegar to the mix. On an empty stomach eat the prunes and drink the liquid. Any cramping simply reduce the prunes. This is an old fashioned folk medicine that works very well.

Pure prune juice may also be effective.

Mineral content: Phosphorus

Iron

Calcium

Potassium

Vitamin content: Vitamin A

Vitamin B Group

Vitamin C

Other nutrients: Oxalic acid

PUMPKIN SEEDS AND PUMPKIN *–Cucurbita pepo*

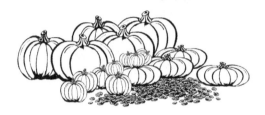

▶ Pumpkin Seeds -

Pumpkin seeds are used in the treatment of expelling intestinal worms.

Pumpkin seeds are known to be an all round nutritional substance with an ability to remove internal parasites. The seeds create an environment in which the parasites cannot live.

Pumpkin seeds are an excellent food to help combat stress due to their mineral and vitamin content that support the body in times of stress.

Mineral content: Phosphorus

Iron

Calcium

Vitamin content: Vitamin A

                        Vitamin B Groups

▶ Pumpkin -

This vegetable is one of the best sources of Vitamin A and provides a healing benefit to conditions affecting the skin and mucous membranes.

Pumpkin also helps to combat infection.

Very nutritious as part of recovery from illness. Iron assists the constitution and this makes pumpkin a significant medicine as part of recovery.

Mineral content: Silicon

                        Potassium

                        Chlorine

                        Sulphur

                        Iron

Vitamin content: Vitamin A

RADISH–*Raphanus gativas*

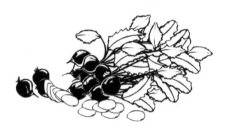

This little bulb type vegetable is packed with health giving properties. Relief can be gained through the use of radish for constipation, runny nose, sore throat, sinusitis, to name a few.

Radish has a mild diuretic action and they can also be useful to add to the diet in the form of juice or whole bulb if fluid retention is a problem.

Eating raw, juiced or blended into smoothies provides opportunities to support wellbeing recovery.

Mineral content: Potassium

Magnesium

Calcium

Iron

Phosphorous

Zinc

Vitamin content: Vitamin C

Vitamin A

Vitamin B

RHUBARB–*Rhuem rhaponticum*

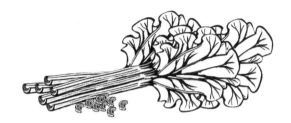

The healing focus of rhubarb is due to the response of the salivary glands as they become stimulated. Saliva is your first laxative and as saliva flows the peristalsis (wave-like contraction from the mouth to the anus) occurs. Through the consumption of rhubarb the bowel is supported to perform. The fibre found in the rhubarb is Excellent to aid the bowel as well as assisting to reduce cholesterol (LDL bad guy).

Rhubarb may irritate if there is inflammatory conditions present such as arthritis due to the oxalic acid.

Mineral content: Iron

Phosphorous

	Potassium
	Calcium
Vitamin content:	Vitamin C
	Vitamin A
	Vitamin B
Other nutrients:	Oxalic acid

ROLLED *OATS –Avena sativa*

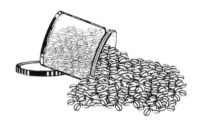

Rolled oats: *houses a broad matrix of minerals and is a general nutritional substance

*improves energy levels

*has a complex chemistry but its main support is provided to the nervous system.

Mineral content: Calcium

Silicon

Iron

Potassium

Sodium

Phosphorus

Vitamin content: Vitamin B Complex

Vitamin B1 - high

Inositol

Oat Milk Recipe

Ingredients: 1 cup of rolled oats 1 litre of cold water

Method: Place ingredients into a container and leave over night in the fridge. Strain and drink throughout the day. Save the oats and use as a cereal.

SORRELL–*Rumex 2acetosa*

The consumption of sorrel has been known to provide the body with much needed vitamins.

Sorrel: *assists in increasing energy

*is a digestive aid

*acts as a mild diuretic, particularly if you drink a broth made with the root.

*is excellent for convalescence by providing valuable energy and vitamins and therefore aiding recovery.

A poultice of the leaves of the sorrel aids 'speedy healing of boils and sebaceous cysts'. (Valnet (1975) Heal Yourself with Vegetables, Fruits and Grains, pg. 181.) Valnet suggests that the drinking of a bouillon made using sorrel can be used as an effective laxative. He also suggests that this formula may be used for pus forming skin infections. (Refer to a modification of Valnet's recipe given at the bottom of this page.)

● **CAUTIONS to be aware of before eating sorrel:**

▶ It is important to note that sorrel is high in oxalate which is a component of kidney stones. Drink a lot of water.

▶ Never take sorrel internally if you suffer from:

> Lung disease

> Asthma at time of attack

> A sensitive stomach

> Arthritis

> Gout

> Kidney stones

Mineral content: Iron

Phosphates

Vitamin content: Vitamin C

Other nutrients: Chlorophyll

Sorrel Bouillon Recipe

Ingredients: 40 gms. Sorrel

20 gms. Lettuce

20 gms. Leek

5 gms. Butter

750 mls. Water

Method: Melt butter in saucepan and place in vegetables. Saute for a few minutes and then add water. Bring to the boil and allow to simmer for a short while. Strain and allow to cool.

SPROUTS

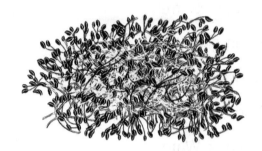

Sprouts come in many varieties. They have been acknowledged by generations over thousands of years to be highly nutritious and a valuable healing food. The simplicity of preparing sprouts could not be easier. Simply take a glass jar, add the seeds and fresh water then let nature perform magic. Seeds by themselves do not have the powerful healing ability as the sprouts, add water allow to germinate and a powerhouse of healing is ready to work for you.

Leslie and Susannah Kenton, in their exceptional book *Raw Energy* (1984) offer 'Sprouts contain a complex array of nutrients and are an excellent source of amino acids, fatty acids and natural sugars, plus a high content of minerals, sprouts are capable of sustaining life on their own, provided several kinds are eaten together' (p. 103).

List of sprouts offered can be mixed and matched to suit the palate. The main thing to consider is to blend several together to achieve maximum benefits.

> Alfalfa
> Chick peas
> Mung beans
> Barley
> Fenugreek
> Lentils
> Mustard
> Oats
> Pumpkin seeds
> Sesame seeds
> Sunflower seeds

This list is not exhaustive and many more can be tried and tested.

STAWBERRIES–Fragaria *ananassa*

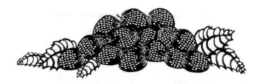

Strawberries may provide skin reactions in some people so be cautious about eating too many (although may be hard to do as they are delicious). Strawberries offer blood cleansing, reduction of gout symptoms, aids in the management of constipation, reduce high blood pressure and reduces catarrh.

To enhance the healing ability of strawberries clinical observation support the effectiveness of strawberries by adding a sprinkle of apple cider vinegar. The two blend well together to activate healing.

Mineral content: Calcium

Iron

Phosphorous

Potassium

Vitamin content: Vitamin C

Vitamin A

Vitamin B

Other nutrients: Lycopene is a powerful antioxidant,

assisting to decrease cell damage,

according to the American Cancer

Society

SWEET POTATO–*Batatas batatas*

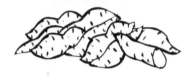

Sweet potato has healing benefits to aid recovery from exercise, assist the bowel in particular where inflammation is present and a bowel balancer to regulate constipation or diarrhoea.

Mineral content: Calcium

Iron

Phosphorous

Potassium

Vitamin content: Vitamin C

Vitamin A

Vitamin B

Other nutrients: Lycopene is a powerful antioxidant, as-sisting to decrease cell damage accord-ing to the American Cancer Society

SPINACH–*Spinacia oleracea*

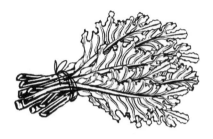

The healing benefits of spinach has been known throughout the world since time immemorial. Literally every system of the body can benefit with the introduction of spinach into the daily diet. Include baby spinach as well.

The powerful antioxidants provide the healing stimulus, supported by a wide range of other minerals and vitamins. Lightly steam or add raw to juices and smoothies will offer wellbeing recovery in a short space of time.

Mineral content: Zinc

Magnesium

Manganese

Iron

Potassium

Calcium

Phosphorous

Folate

Vitamin content: Vitamin C

Vitamin K

Vitamin A

Vitamin B

Vitamin E

Other nutrients: Chlorophyll

Lutein

Zeaxanthin

TOMATO–*Solanum lycopersicum*

The readily available tomato has excited scientists over the past decade as it offers a very powerful nutrient called lycopene. This is what provides the red colour to the fruit and a major healing element.

Tomato is a heart tonic and also a blood tonic

Mineral content: Calcium

Iron

Magnesium

Manganese

Phosphorous

Zinc

Vitamin content: Vitamin C

Vitamin A

Vitamin E

Vitamin K

Other nutrients: Lycopene is a powerful antioxidant, assisting to decrease cell damage. According to the American Cancer Society observation of populations who have increased consumption of lycopene through tomatoes appear to have lower risk of cancer.

Fibre assisting to lower cholesterol

◑ **Note**

Caution: Suffers of arthritis and inflammatory conditions note they cannot eat tomatoes, eggplants or potatoes.

TURNIP -*Brassica napus*

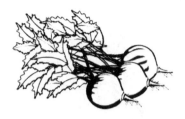

It is the top of the turnip that is very nutritious.

Turnip juice is very high in vitamins and minerals

Turnip is nutritionally balanced.

Mineral content: Magnesium

Iron

Sulphur

Copper

Iodine

Vitamin content: Vitamin A

Vitamin C

Vitamin B Complex

WATERCRESS - *Nasturtium officinale*

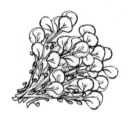

Watercress is a very nutritious food and as a medicine shines to aid many conditions. Ancient Chinese medicine find the use of watercress to assist the dysfunctions in the mouth such as mouth ulcers. Watercress is also an excellent digestive aid and blood purifier.

Mineral content: Potassium

Sodium

Iron

Magnesium

Vitamin content: Vitamin C

Vitamin A

Vitamin D

Vitamin B-6

Vitamin B – 12

Other nutrients: Chlorophyll

WATERMELON–*Cucurbita citrullus*

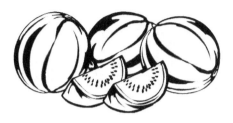

Historically this fruit is reported to be of value in treating abnormal kidney conditions.

The fruit is an excellent source of moisture for the body aiding a healthy urinary tract. It is an effective diuretic.

Mineral content: Iron

Calcium

Potassium

Phosphorus

Vitamin content: Vitamin A

Vitamin B Group

Vitamin C

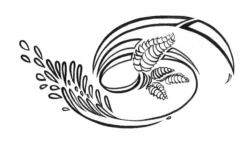

Section Three
Nutritional Elements

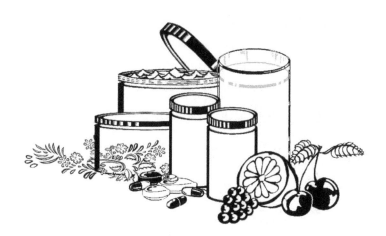

VITAMINS, MINERALS AND OTHER NUTRIENTS

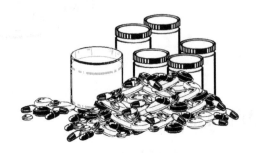

Vitamins:

A

Acts as an anti-oxidant.

Aids healing of the skin.

Strengthens cartilage and bone.

Acts as a growth vitamin.

Benefits the intestines.

Heals mucosa

Aids sleep patterns.

Benefits the arteries.

Excellent for the eyes.

Aids management of PMT symptoms.

Assists with the treatment of fatigue.

The dose range is very important as it may prove toxic in large doses.

A - Carotene

Recent research has shown that Carotene works as a protection against cancer. This is still under intensive research.

Transfers to Vitamin A when in the body.

Biotin

A water soluble vitamin.

Produced by intestinal bacteria.

Deficiencies are rare but may lead to depression and or mild anaemia.

It should be noted that the eating of raw egg white can contribute to a deficiency.

Within the egg white there is a protein called Avidin. When combined with Biotin a compound is formed that cannot be absorbed. Cooking the egg destroys the action of Avidin. (Diet with Vitamins, pg.76.)

Increased amounts of Biotin are recommended during anti-biotic treatment. Has been found to be useful for skin conditions.

Research indicates that the introduction of Biotin has been used to prevent cot death. (Diet With Vitamins, pg. 32.)

Essential for the maintenance of healthy skin, hair, sweat glands, nerves, bone marrow and the glands producing sex hormones.

B Complex (B Group)

Provides the body with energy

Aids growth.

Excellent during convalescence.

Aids metabolism.

Assists with the management of pain.

Treatment for inflamed gums.

Aids treatment of irritability.

Aids adrenal gland function.

Assists with the management of constipation.

B1 - Thiamine

Assists the body to utilise energy from carbohydrates.

Assists growth of young children.

Required for mental alertness.

Increase your B1 intake when suffering with a fever.

Increase your intake of B1 during pregnancy and lactation.

Essential for the health of the entire nervous system.

Common symptoms of deficiency of B1 is depression, anxiety and nervousness.

Low Vitamin B1 can also result in shortness of breath and irregular heart beat.

B1 is lost in the cooking process. The body is depleted of this vitamin through the drinking of alcohol.

B2 - Riboflavin

The appetite vitamin.

This vitamin promotes digestion and growth.

Lack of Vitamin B2 has been found to be responsible for eye fatigue.

A gritty feeling in the eyes.

Splits in the comer of the mouth.

Some laboratory investigations have revealed that large quantities of Brewer's Yeast, which contains

Riboflavin protected laboratory animals from liver cancer. (The Complete Home Guide To All Vitamins, pg. 121)

B3 - Niacin

Assists in energy production.

Improves blood circulation.

Assists in the balancing of fat levels in blood.

Aids the digestive process.

Assists hormone production.

Deficiency signs: mental depression, digestive disturbances, personality changes, mental disorders, general fatigue, muscular weakness or skin allergies.

B5 - Pantothenic Acid

This is a water soluble vitamin.

Pantothenic Acid is unstable when exposed to heat.

It is essential for the formation of anti-bodies and

therefore useful for the health of the immune system.

Our ability to mobilise carbohydrates is assisted by this vitamin Vital for healthy nerves and skin.

Essential for the maintenance of blood sugar levels.

Regarded as an anti-stress vitamin. Research is underway to investigate the possibility that B5 may produce an anticarcinogenic reaction as well as assisting the function of the pancreas for the treatment of marginal diabetics. (Robert Benowicz,Vitamins and You)

B6 - Pyridoxine

Known as Pyridoxine, Pyridoxal or Pyridoxamine.

This vitamin is often referred to as the anti-depressant vitamin.

Common symptoms of Vitamin B6 deficiency are:

Scaly dry skin around the eyes

Scaly dry skin around the nose or mouth

Splitting lips

Inflammation of the tongue

Migraines

Breast discomfort

Irritability or swollen fingers and ankles associated with premenstrual syndrome. Muscle pain

Joint pain

Carpal tunnel syndrome

Fatigue

Increased amounts of Vitamin B6 should be consumed by women taking the contraceptive pill and persons who consume alcohol and/or smoke. This vitamin can be used as a mild diuretic.

B12 - Cobalamin

Assists with anaemia.

Assists with pain relief.

Assists with rheumatic pain.

Aids the treatment of colitis.

Aids the treatment of allergies.

Assists in the management of fatigue.

C - Ascorbic Acid

A major assimilator for Iron.

Assists the immune system.

Assists with both physical and mental exhaustion.

Aids in the treatment of allergies.

Aids treatment of skin conditions.

Aids reduction of cholesterol.

Antioxidant.

D - Calciferol

The sunlight vitamin.

Regulates all mineral and vitamin metabolism, especially Calcium and Phosphorus.

Vitamin D is better described as a hormone.

This vitamin is required by the thyroid to manufacture hormones.

Assists with the growth, maintenance and repair of the bones.

In combination with Vitamin A, wards off colds and flu.

E - Tocopherol

Generally excellent for the treatment of reproductive disorders.

Assists in the treatment of impoteney.

Assists with retarded genital development.

Aids in the treatment of period pain.

Aids in the treatment of menopausal symptoms.

Aids in the treatment of nerve pain.

Aids in the treatment of arteriosclerosis.

Aids in the treatment of skin conditions.

Aids in the treatment of leg ulcers.

Antioxidant.

G - Refer B2

Inositol

This is a soluble member of the vitamin B family, although not really considered a true Vitamin.

Inositol is produced from glucose by intestinal bacteria.

Deficiency signs are mild anxiety, unhealthy hair, or high cholesterol.

Although this is not the only Vitamin responsible for these symptoms, by including more cereal and fresh vegetables in your diet, will help combat the possibility of a deficiency. This Vitamin is stable during the cooking process. Interestingly inositol prevents the accumulation of fats in the liver and other organs.

K - Phylloquinone (Natural K)

Assists in the treatment of hepatitis.

Assists in the treatment of jaundice.

Assists in the treatment of colitis.

Assists in the treatment of skin disorders.

Assists in the treatment of chilblains.

Assists in the manufacture of components.

Crucial to blood clotting to prevent bleeding.

This vitamin is found in dark leafy green vegetables, alfalfa and kelp.

P - Bioflavonoids

This vitamin is found in fresh fruit and vegetables.

Enhances the action of Vitamin C.

The blend of Vitamin C and P is beneficial in the management of rheumatism.

Vitamin P assists in the management of arthritis, ulcers, high cholesterol and the common cold.

U

Recently it has been discovered that Vitamin U is useful in the healing of ulcers. "Cabbage which is high in Vitamin U, is a valuable vegetable to assist with the management of leg ulcers.

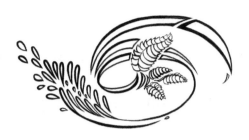

Minerals:

Calcium

Assists in the building of healthy bones.

Assists in the growth of healthy teeth.

Assists in the healing of wounds.

Assists to offset the effect of acidic conditions.

Provides the body with the strength and endurance for daily activity.

Important for healthy muscle tone.

Tones and strengthens the heart muscle.

Assists the clotting factor of the blood.

Assists in balancing metabolism

Chlorine

Assists with the digestion of food.

Chlorine is found within the fluid of the brain, assisting to protect the brain and spinal cord.

Combines with potassium and sodium to maintain fluid balance.

Most foods have some amount of chlorine in them.

Chromium

Protein around the bloodstream.

Is a trace mineral.

Is used for the transportation of glucose.

Is beneficial in reducing sugar cravings.

Cobalt

Cobalt is required in small amounts in the body as it is a component of Vitamin B12, which in turn is needed for the formation of healthy red blood cells and the formation of myelin nerve coverings.

Assists in the treatment of anaemic states.

Copper

Aids in red blood cell regeneration and may prevent nutritional anaemia.

Deficiency is rare, in fact, an excess is more common.

Iodine

Iodine is necessary for the growth of children.

It regulates the thyroid gland.

Assists in burning of excess fat.

A deficiency may lead to irregular heart beat, hardening of the arteries, dry hair or poor mental abilities.

Iron

At least a quarter of the iron that comes into our body is derived from meat. There are however a number of vegetables that offer a reasonable amount of iron,

Globe artichoke is one.

Absorption of Iron is varied and very important. Most foods that have Iron also contain Phosphates as these are complementary to the absorption ratio of the iron. Vitamin C is a major assimilator for Iron and Iron rich foods generally house vitamin C.

Iron aids in red blood cell regeneration and can assist to prevent nutritional anaemia.

Improves energy.

Magnesium

Assists the nervous system.

Assists with the production of energy.

Promotes a restful sleep.

Promotes a healthy complexion.

Considered to be of vital importance to the function of the heart.

Considered to be a key anti-stress mineral.

Relaxes stressed muscles.

Assists with the management of PMS.

Manganese

Essential for healthy joint development.

Assists in the treatment of eczema

Deficiency may produce heart conditions.

Essential for effective digestion.

Nickel

Assists the body to utilise sugar.

Potassium

Assists to strengthen the heart.

Assists with muscle related problems.

Assists in helping to maintain fluid balance when combined with chlorine and sodium.

Phosphorus

Promotes mental alertness.

Nourishes the brain.

Assists in the growth and development of bones.

Assists in the growth of healthy hair.

Assists in the growth of healthy teeth.

Assists in the relief of fatigue.

Assists in the treatment of eczema.

Selenium

Biologically it is very similar to Vitamin E.

Several studies have shown that Selenium possesses definite anti-cancer characteristics. Some suspect that among other things Selenium helps by slowing down cancer at its very earliest stages, permitting cells to heal themselves before they are taken over by the cancer process.' (Mark Bricklin, Natural Healing - A Complete A To Z Guide For Australians)

Studies conducted on laboratory animals, where selenium has been introduced into the diet, has reduced the growth rate of tumours.

Silicon

Found mainly in the outer layer of fruits and vegetables

Assists in the cleansing of the blood.

Aids blood circulation.

Assists the hardening of teeth.

Promotes healthy hair.

Beneficial for eyesight.

Beneficial for the skin.

Aids the strengthening of finger nails.

Assists with the treatment of skin rashes.

Sodium

Assists in maintaining fluid balance when combined

with chlorine and potassium.

Sulphur

Assists in the purification of the blood.

Assists is the growth of healthy, glossy hair.

Promotes bile secretion, assisting the digestive process.

Improves the function of the liver.

Assists the body to heal.

Zinc

Assists in the development of healthy bones and teeth.

Zinc is the main healing mineral.

Essential for healthy hair.

Essential for the proper action of insulin.

Essential for the health of the prostate gland.

A deficiency may lead to acne, dermatitis, ulcers, fatigue and susceptibility to infection.

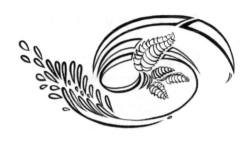

Acids:

Amino Acids - There Are 22 Naturally Occurring Amino Acids.

These acids are the building blocks for protein.

Used in combination these acids may be used to treat a wide range of conditions. Amino acids are generally divided into four categories, essential, semi-essential, non-essential and others. An excellent text that discusses Amino acids in depth is Elson Haas (1992) Staying Healthy with Nutrition

Folic Acid

A water soluble Vitamin in the B Complex group. Foods containing Folic Acid should be consumed by pregnant women.

Green leafy vegetables, avocado, fresh nuts and wheatgerm are good sources of Folic Acid.

A loss of nutrients occurs during heating. Juices or raw food is the best source.

Folic Acid is essential for a healthy nervous system.

Gamma Linolenic Acid

GLA is a dietary omega 6 and is found to be useful in the management of high cholesterol, depression, skin conditions, some menopausal presentations and diabetic neuropathy

Hydrochloric Acid

Combined with Chlorine, in adequate ratio, this acid blends to form the chyme that breaks the food into small passable particles.

Malic Acid

Assists in the neutralising of the by-products of digestion.

Oxalic Acid

Assists the clotting factor of the blood.

Tartaric Acid

Assists in the neutralising of the by products of digestion.

Other nutrients:

Arginine

Antioxidant that offers assistance in restoring tissue throughout the body

Betaine

Aids the digestion of proteins and may reduce food sensitivity.

Asparagine

This is a powerful healer by attaching itself to Vitamin A.

Chlorophyll

Gives plants their green appearance.

Chlorophyll is a blood builder.

Acts as a body cleanser.

Acts as a blood purifier.

Cinarin

Improves liver cell regeneration.

Enzymes

Amylase and Protease assist with the treatment of constipation.

Bromelain - the pineapple enzyme - reduces swelling and inflammation in the soft tissues and joints. Helps in the prevention and treatment of cardiovascular disease.

Carpaine is thought to be helpful for the heart.

Erepsin is an enzyme that assists in the breaking down of protein.

Papain assists with the digestive process and is soothing on the gut.

Essential Oils

The antiseptic action of the aromatic principle found within some plants.

Anethole an anti-fungal and anti-bacterial.

Ficins

Assists the digestive process.

Flavonoids

Antioxidants and are powerful in assisting healing as they have impressive anti-inflammatory action as well as a blend of activities to support the entire body. Flavonoids in many cases provide the colour seen in foods.

Glycerine

This is a commercial preparation purchased in pharmacies.

Useful as a sweetening agent.

Useful as a substance to assist with the adherence of a substance to an anatomical surface.

Glycosides

A chemical with a sugar and non sugar component.

Gum

Gum produces a protective layer for the large intestine.

Histidine

An amino acid offering support for arthritis and inflammatory conditions.

Inulin

Assists in the assimilation process, through the pancreas, to assist the management of diabetes.

Natural Sugars

These occur naturally in the plant kingdom and are present in many fruits and vegetables.

Assist in the production of vital energy.

They provide unprocessed sugar and are more favourable, to be included in the diet, than those highly refined sugars found in isolated forms.

Nerve Salts

These are cell salts that are found in foods and converted through the body and these salts are found to be a nutritional aid for the nervous system.

Pectin

A substance found under the skin of some foods, particularly apples.

Pectin is one of the active constituents that assists in the lowering of cholesterol and providing regular bowel actions.

Plant Estrogens

Natural substances in plants that facilitate an hormonal reaction.

Punicalagin

A powerful antioxidant found in the pomegranate

Section Four
Herbal Teas Beverages
And Spices

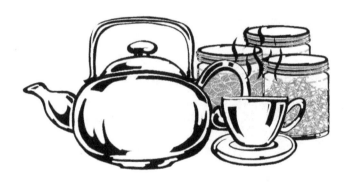

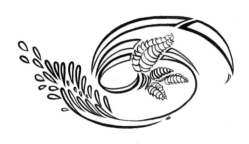

Alfalfa tea

Purchase from your local super market or your health food store.

Aniseed tea

Purchase from your local supermarket or health food store.

Apple cider and ginger beverage

Ingredients: 500mls of apple cider vinegar

3 tablespoons of freshly grated ginger

Method: To 500mls of Apple Cider Vinegar add 3 teaspoons of freshly grated ginger. Allow to rest for 1 day. Take 10mls x 2 day in 50mls of water. Eating the grated ginger works well.

Apple cider vinegar, ginger and peppermint beverage

Ingredients: 500mls of apple cider vinegar

3 tablespoons of freshly grated ginger

1 cup of fresh peppermint or common mint leaves

Method: To 500mls of Apple Cider Vinegar add 3 teaspoons of freshly grated ginger and mint leaves. Allow to rest for 1 day. Take 10mls x 2 day in 50mls of water. Eating the grated ginger works well.

Apple cider and lemon tea

Ingredients: 1 tablespoon of Apple Cider Vinegar must be unfiltered and has Mother in it. Read the label.

Juice of ½ a lemon.

Small amount of water (hot or cold).

Method: Mix and drink.

Apple peel tea

Ingredients: Apple peel

Method: Lay the peels on a rack and dry them, allow air to flow through rack. When they are very brittle, using a pestle and mortar, powder the peel. Put one teaspoon in a cup of boiling water and drink.

Black currant tea

Ingredients: 2 tablespoons of black currants

Method: Pour hot water over the currants using a coffee mug. Cover and allow to steep for 30minutes. Drink the liquid and eat the currants.

Blackberry tea

Ingredients: 1 teaspoon of whole fruit.

1 cup of hot water.

Method: Pulp the fruit. Allow the fruit to infuse in the hot water and drink.

Blackberry leaf tea

Ingredients: 1 teaspoon of dried or fresh leaves.

1 cup of boiling water.

Method: Steep leaves in boiling water and drink.

Caraway seed tea

Purchase from your local supermarket or health food store.

Alternatively take 1 tablespoon of seeds and add 1 cup of boiling water. Allow to steep for 20 minutes. Consume liquid and eat the seeds.

Chamomile tea

Purchase from your local supermarket or health food store, or grow you own

Coriander as a spice

Use the fresh leaves and stalks and or the powdered seeds.

Corn silk tea

Purchase from your local supermarket or health food store, or grow your own corn and use the silk.

Couch-grass tea

Purchase from your local supermarket or health food store.

Dandelion root tea

Purchase from your local supermarket, health food store, or grow your own.

Fennel tea

Purchase from your local supermarket, health food store, or grow your own.

Fenugreek tea

Purchase from your local supermarket, health food store.

Gin-soaked raisin remedy

This remedy is under teas as I did not know where else to put it. Several clients reported being introduced to this remedy and was not sure of the source. I found it in Joan and Lydia Wilen's book *Healing Remedies. Enjoy*

Ingredients: 500 gms golden or black raisins

500mls Gin

Method: Use a glass pyrex dish and have ready a glass jar with tight lid

Spread the golden or black raisins in the dish and cover with the gin. Cover with a cloth and leave them until all the gin is absorbed, usually 5 days or so. Over this time toss the fruit to get the gin wrapped around them. Once all the gin has been absorbed transfer the fruit to the jar and place on lid.

Do not refrigerate.

Each day have 9 (only nine as you may be tempted to have more). Usually with breakfast or place in any of the smoothies or juices.

This may take days to months to work, yet reports indicate impressive results.

Ginger tea

Ingredients: 1 teaspoon of fresh, grated ginger.

1 cup of boiling water.

Method: Place the grated ginger into a cup and pour boiling water over it. Allow to draw for ten minutes. Strain and drink.

or

Purchase from your local supermarket or health food store.

Ginger and lemon tea

Ingredients: 1 teaspoon of fresh, grated ginger.

Juice of ½ lemon

1 teaspoon of grated lemon rind

1 cup of boiling water.

Method: Place the grated ginger, lemon juice and peel into a cup and pour boiling water over it. Cover and allow to draw for ten minutes. Strain and drink. Eat the ginger and lemon rind.

Green bean pod tea

Ingredients: 1 teaspoon of bean pods (remove from green beans)

1 cup of boiling water.

Method: Take the pods of the bean and place 1 teaspoon in a cup and pour boiling water over them. Allow to draw for ten minutes. Strain and drink, eat the pods.

Hawthorn berry tea

Purchase from your local supermarket or health food store.

Hops

Purchase from your local supermarket or health food store.

Jasmine tea

Purchase from your local health food shop.

Lemon balm tea

Ingredients: 10 lemon balm leaves.

1 cup of boiling water.

Method: Take the leaves and place in a cup and pour boiling water over them. Allow to draw for ten minutes. Strain and drink.

Purchase from your local health food store or grow your own plant

Oatmilk

Ingredients Rolled oats and water

Method: One cup of rolled oats to one litre of cold water, let stand for a few hours, strain (refrigerate unused portion) will last for several days. May be refrigerated during the drawing process.

Loquat leaf tea

Ingredients: 3 dried loquat leaves (make sure fine hair have been removed)

1 cup of boiling water.

Method: Take the leaves and place in a cup and pour boiling water over them. Allow to draw for ten minutes. Strain and drink.

Meadowsweet tea

Purchase from your local supermarket or health food store.

Onion syrup

Ingredients: 3 large brown or white onions

1 tray

Cling wrap

Honey

Method: Finely slice the onions and line the bottom of the tray

Cover with a fine layer of honey

Cover the tray with cling wrap

Refrigerate overnight

The following day separate the onion syrup and strain off.

For children 1 teaspoon x 2 day and adults 1 tablespoon x 2 to 3 x a day

Parsley tea

Ingredients: 1 teaspoon of dried parsley.

1 cup of boiling water.

Method: Place the dried parsley into a cup and pour boiling water over it. Allow to draw for ten minutes. Strain and drink.

or

Purchase from the spice section of the super-market or grow your own.

Peppermint tea

Ingredients: 2 teaspoons of dried peppermint leaves.

1 cup of boiling water.

Method: Place the dried peppermint leaves into a cup and pour boiling water over it. Allow to draw for ten minutes. Strain and drink.

or

Purchase from your local supermarket, health food store, or grow your own.

Raspberry leaf tea

Purchase from your local supermarket or health food store.

Sage tea

Purchase from your local supermarket, health food

store, or grow your own

Slippery elm tea

Ingredients: 1 teaspoon of Slippery Elm Powder.

200 mls of warm water.

Method: Mix powder and water slowly adding water as the product expands and drink.

Purchase from your local health food store.

Thyme tea

Purchase from your local supermarket, health food store, or grow your own.

Walnut tea

Ingredients: 10 shelled walnuts and water

Method: Place ten walnuts in a mug of boiling water, seal top of mug, let cool for ten minutes then strain and drink. Eat walnuts.

Watermelon seed tea

Ingredients: Dried watermelon seeds.

1 cup of hot water.

Method: Crush 2 teaspoons of dried watermelon seeds and steep in a cup of hot water for one hour. Stir and drain. Drink a cup of this tea four times daily.

Collect the seeds from a watermelon and air dry them.

Yarrow tea

Purchase from your local supermarket, health food store, or grow your own.

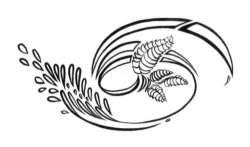

Section Five
Oil Treatments

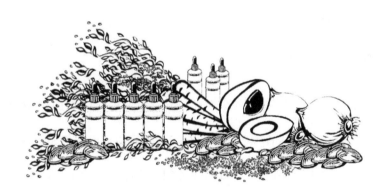

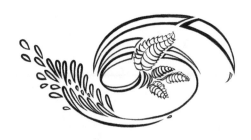

OIL TREATMENTS

Avocado oil

Avocado oil, is useful as a food for the skin.

Avocado oil contains vitamins, proteins and fatty acids.

It may be blended with carrot oil for the management of dry skin, particularly eczema or psoriasis. Where there is an inflammatory condition of the skin, blend Avocado and Almond Oil in equal parts and apply direct to affected area.

Avocado oil may be purchased from a health food store.

Cabbage ointment

Maybe available at healthfood stores

Alternatively blend 20mls of cabbage juice into 60grms of vegetable sorbalene

Carrot oil

Carrot Oil contains a blend of minerals, vitamins and healing agents.

Carrot Oil may be used for skin healing and in the treatment of conjunctivitis and styes. Itching of the skin, eczema and the reduction of scarring are all indications for the use of Carrot Oil.

A blend of almond or olive oil with Carrot Oil is useful for dry skin. Use a ratio of 1 part carrot to 10 parts almond or olive oil.

Carrot Oil may be purchased from a health food store.

Coconut oil

Must be virgin and cold pressed.

Coconut oil is an excellent oil to address dry skin and may be added to a vegetable sorbalene.

Is a great taste so have a tablespoon a day to help dry skin.

Lavender oil

Lavender Oil is an essential oil and is useful for treating many conditions. Additionally it is useful in the home as a general disinfectant.

Lavender Oil has been most favoured throughout time as a treatment for burns and scalds. It is most effective if directly applied to the skin. By applying a small amount to acne spots they will dry up and the antiseptic and antibiotic content will assist with the healing. Blended with Almond Oil, in a ratio of 1 part Lavender and 10 parts Almond, this oil is very useful for the healing of wounds and to avoid scarring. Lavender Oil is also regarded as an anti-depressant and has been found useful for this condition.

The list of healing abilities of Lavender Oil appears to be endless:

Acne/undiluted

Burns/Undiluted

Infections/Undiluted

Bacterial conditions/Undiluted

Sores/Undiluted

Cuts/Undiluted

Inflammation of the skin/add almond or avocado

Eczema/add almond or avocado

Dermatitis/add almond or avocado

Lavender Oil can be purchased from a health food store. Ensure it is labelled, as Pure Essential Lavender Oil.

Be aware of synthetic and cheap imitations.

Muscular Oil Combination

Both of the oil combinations, listed below, are effective treatments for muscular aches and pains.

Blend: 10 drops of Rosemary Oil.

6 drops of Lemon grass Oil.

9 drops of Juniper Oil.

Add the above oils to 50mls. of Almond Oil and massage the affected area.(Aromatherapy for Everyone, Tisserand, p. 203.)

Or

Blend: 10 drops Lavender Oil

5 drops Rosemary Oil

15 drops Cypress Oil.

Add the above oils to 50mls of Almond Oil and massage the affected area.

(The Fragrant Pharmacy, Valerie Ann Wormwood, p.105)

All the oils used in the combination blends may be purchased from a health food store. Ensure they are pure essential oils.

Onion oil

This oil is a powerful healer for the ears. If you are un-sure of the cause I of an ear ache then you should con-sult your doctor before using any treatment. Onion Oil is excellent for ear ache associated with excess wax. Apply 3 drops of the warmed oil into the ear and place a cotton wool wad in the ear to prevent leakage from the ear. The oil may be refrigerated and rewarmed by heating a spoon in boiling water and place the oil on the hot spoon. Allow the oil to gently warm from the heat of the spoon. Always test the temperature.

◑ **CAUTION: Warm and not hot oil.**

To extract the oil

Ingredients: 1 onion.

water.

Method: Take the onion DO NOT PEEL IT. Suspend the onion over water in a heated oven until the onion is soft. This can be done by placing the onion on a rack in the oven, and suspending it over a tray of water on a lower rack. The steam will cook the onion. Once the onion is soft, and cooled place it in a clean cloth and twist to draw the onion oil from the flesh of the vegetable. DO NOT PEEL at any time.

Sweet almond oil

Sweet Almond Oil is used as a base, or carry oil. It is excellent for all skin conditions and is suitable for all skin types. It is used for its ability to address dryness of the skin and where there is inflammation or general skin soreness.

Sweet Almond Oil is nutritionally beneficial for the skin due to a high vitamin, mineral and protein content.

The oil is obtained from the kernel of the almond.

Sweet Almond Oil can be purchased from a health food store.

Tea tree oil

Tea Tree Oil is a general, all round healer with a particular focus on fungal conditions around the body. It is also an anti-viral and anti-bacterial formula.

Ringworm can be treated with this oil, as can tinea. The oil is safe to use undiluted and applied directly to the skin. The inhalation of the oil for infected sinuses can be complementary to your health care management. Place 10 drops into boiling water and inhale the steam. This is also very useful for relief when suffering from the common cold.

Tea Tree Oil can be purchased from a health food store.

Thyme oil

Thyme Oil is an essential oil and is an anti fungal preparation that is useful in addressing stubborn cases of tinea.

Is a powerful anti—viral, anti-biotic and antiseptic agent to be applied externally.

It may be sprinkled around the house as an insect repellent.

Thyme Oil can be purchased from a health food store.

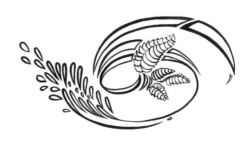

Section Six
Juices And Smoothies

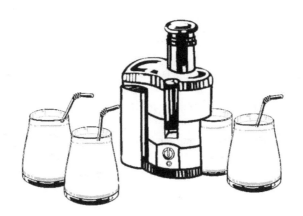

First and most importantly always ensure you dilute the juice down with either water, oat −milk, almond milk or rice milk .

Juices and smoothies have become quite trendy and popular and as usual the marketing hype that goes with the fads can be downright unhealthy. To address 'convenience' an example of this is to purchase vegetable powders to add to juices and smoothies.

Better still why not go to the fruit and vegetable market and buy the real thing? Now that is a unique idea! Please steer away from pills and potions and only use when directed to by a qualified practitioner. Choose fresh fruit and vegetables and support the growers while we still have them.

One important consideration when making juices and smoothies is to be aware of the nutrients that are in the products and always consider the less is more concept. Smaller amounts are much better than a lot of product.

In the following combinations you will note the amount of product and quantity of product is quite low. This is due to the powerhouse of nutrition that is found within the products. Small amounts over a longer period is better than a large amount over a short period where your body struggles to assimilate the dense nutrients.

FAQ's	
Is a smoothie or juice better?	Either, however the smoothie will be blended and have the fibre included and yoghurt or milk blended.
Should I take some of the fibre when I juice and include it in my diet?	Yes. In that way you are getting the fibre that is so good to help cleanse.
Can I have too much fibre?	Yes. Make sure you have regular intake of fibre yet drink a good amount of water and ensure the fibre is hydrated. If having oats for breakfast soak them overnight as an example to ensure good hydration.

I started on smoothies when I purchased a blender and added chia seeds but I am constipated and feel unwell.	This is not uncommon as the suggested blends have too much of a good thing; also the chia seeds are very gelatinous and become hard to digest in large amounts. Less is more and always soak the seeds for a few hours first.
Can I have too many smoothies or juices?	Yes. The nutrition in the foods is very high and quite complex. They are powerful healing medicines and should be treated with great respect. So have less. Even diluting them with 50% water is a good idea to work out your specific balance as everyone is different.
Can I mix and match whatever I like?	Yes, however work on the 1 fruit and 3 vegetable rule to start with as that is a good balance. If you are treating a particular condition then follow the recommendations.
I started on lots of fresh fruit smoothies and juices but found my skin broke out and I developed lots of pimples.	This is not uncommon as the high fructose levels can do this. Although good medicine, too much is not effective. Try 1 fruit and 3 vegetables as a balance.

What is good to add to the fruit and vegetables to make a smoothie?	Rice, Goat or Almond milk or a natural unsweetened yoghurt.
Can I really stimulate healing simply by eating more fruit and vegetables, sprouts, nuts and seeds?.	Most definitely as they house powerful healing agents. When combined and blended correctly people report they can actually feel them working as they enter the body.

Blends

BLEND	WHY USE
Energiser Carrot ½ Apple and peel ½ Lettuce ¼ (any)	Energises the body. Good for recovery from conditions. When a bounce-back is needed.
Internal cleanser 3 outer leaves of cabbage ¼ beetroot and leaves ½ carrot	Internal cleansing of the body. Following food poisoning or any condition particularly that affects the stomach, urinary tract or the bowel.
Immune booster ½ apple ½ beetroot and leaves 2 pomegranates 1 radish	Immune booster to build, strengthen and tone the immune system
Digestive aid 1 handful of watercress 1 handful of peppermint leaves ½ carrot ½ apple 1 teaspoon apple cider vinegar	Digestive aid is a balancing combination to assist to soothe and settle an upset digestive system. Nervy or stressed and tummy becomes upset

Immune activator 1 apple 1 carrot ½ lemon plus peel ½ orange plus peel 2 cabbage leaves	Early signs of a cold hit the body with the immune activator
Immune support ½ carrot ½ apple 2 radish ½ lemon plus peel Small handful of water-cress	Immune support is called upon when the cold has taken hold and you need to have support for the system. In particular when the cold activates painful and sore throat.
Skin cleanser ¼ beetroot ½ apple 3 leaves cabbage	Skin cleanser is a good balance between blood cleansing and a liver tonic.
Blood tonic 1 cup of mixed berries 1 carrot ¼ beetroot 1 teaspoon apple cider vinegar ½ pomegranate	Blood tonic is a great pick – you – up and really hits the spot if you have been ill and need to get the bounce back in your step.

Lung cleanser 1 3 outer leaves cabbage or bok choy ½ carrot Thumb size piece of horseradish	Lung cleanser (1) is like a pipe cleaner and works very well.
Lung cleanser 2 2 radish 1 apple 2 outer leaves of cabbage ½ cup alfalfa sprouts	Lung cleanser (2) is an alternative to lung cleanser (2) offering a choice.
Heart support (1) 1 apple ½ cup mixed berries Fresh ginger to taste (if you are not used to ginger then start with a tiny amount and work up ½ tomato Pinch of chilli (optional)	Heart support (1) is a fantastic combination and works very well. Full of nutrients the heart loves and assisted with ginger to get the circulation moving is fantastic.

Heart support (2) ½ Cucumber 1 apple ¼ capsicum red or green Juice of 1 pomegranate	Heart support (2) is a balanced blend of nutrition that supports the heart. Mix and match with the above blend.
Energy booster 1 carrot 1 apple ½ cup watercress	Energy booster activates energy and works very well. There can be no healing without energy and this is a simple yet powerful combination.
Wellbeing recovery tonic Pinch of chilli (Optional) 1 carrot ½ apple Ginger to taste	Improving the circulation and stimulating the flow of blood assists here and this recovery tonic is palatable and one of the most popular.
Liver tonic ¼ raw beetroot Juice of 1 pomegranate	The liver is a very important organ and this blend supports the liver to perform to its optimum.

Fluid remover ½ cup of watermelon + seeds (if lucky enough to find them) 2 stalks of celery Handful of fresh parsley	Fluid remover works well when taken daily
Muscle health (1) 1 carrot 1 apple ½ banana 3 leaves of celery Muscle health (2) 2 stalks celery ½ carrot ½ cup broccoli	The muscles of the body pro- vide the ability to move and movement is essential to acti- vate wellbeing.

Bowel health (1)

½ mango
4 figs fresh or reconstituted (place the dried figs in a cup of water)

Bowel health (2)

½ mango
3 cabbage or spinach leaves
⅛th teaspoon of bi-carb soda
¼ beetroot

Bowel health (3)

½ mango
3 figs (dried or fresh) if dried soak overnight in water
1 pear
¼ cup cauliflower

The bowel is so important as the better the bowel functions the healthier you feel. Focus on getting good elimination on a regular basis and you have the potential to achieve a sense of wellbeing.

Immune support
Viral invader
¼ raw onion
2 radish
3 cabbage leaves
Handful sprouts (any)
Pinch powdered clove

Immune support
Viral destroyer
Not for the faint hearted
¼ raw onion
 2 cabbage leaves
1 radish
1 apple
½ carrot
½ roasted lemon + peel

Immune health
tonic (1)
½ apple
2 radish
¼ onion
2 leaves cabbage
½ red capsicum
½ roasted lemon
Pinch of chilli (optional)

Immune health
tonic (2)
¼ fresh pineapple
ginger (fresh) to taste
¼ cup cauliflower
Pinch black pepper or
chilli

The immune system is the core to the entire body. Helping to support the immune system activates its ability to protect you as you are challenged with all the invaders that lurk out there.

The combinations on offer here, although a taste challenge, can assist the immune system to spring into action.

Take small amounts across the day instead of trying to get it all down at once.
A shot glass is recommended.

Memory booster ½ tomato ½ apple ½ cup cabbage or kale (lightly steamed) ½ red capsicum ½ cup mixed sprout 2 tablespoons grated fresh ginger	As many people struggle with loss of memory, often it may have more to do with general lack of nutrients coming into the body. This blend is a good start to activate the circulation and help memory.
Arthritis pain reducer 1 carrot ½ lemon + peel 2 stalks of celery including leaves if available ½ cup fresh parsley and or 6 green beans 10mls of apple cider vinegar	As we all age our muscles and bones struggle. Often it is due to lack of balanced nutrients. By combining this blend and linking with bone and muscle health suggestions many have reported outstanding results.

Pain relief ¼ lettuce 6 green beans 3 cabbage leaves ½ cup sprouts (any) 1 stalk celery ½ cup of fresh parsley or 6 green beans Pinch of chilli (optional)	When pain strikes and pain killers may be slow to work, this blend is a balance of nutrients to aid in pain reduction.
Tummy soother (1) ½ cup peppermint or common mint leaves 1 cup chopped pineapple Thumb size fresh ginger ¼ raw peeled potato Tummy soother (2) ½ cup mint or peppermint leaves 1 cup pineapple ginger to taste ¼ cup of fresh paw paw ⅓ of whole lemon + peel ⅛th teaspoon of bi-carb	The tummy certainly has a lot to do and can produce a lot of pain and discomfort if not working well. These blends assist the digestive process.

Insomnia ⅓ lettuce 1 apple 1 raw egg ½ cup of oatmilk	Restless sleep can leave you feeling run down and out of sorts. Getting a good night sleep is a must as you restore and revitalise.
Nervine tonic ¼ lettuce 1 egg (raw) 1 apple 1 cup of sprouts (any)	In the 21st Century with the fast paced lifestyle many of us have sometimes we need to settle our nerves. This tonic may assist to help settle those jangled nerves.
Good health tonic 1 cup of sprouts (any) 1 apple ½ carrot 1 cup of oat-milk ¼ raw turnip ½ cup fresh parsley Pinch of chilli (optional)	As an all-rounder and just to keep wellbeing going this tonic is full of good nutrition. Use this as a foundation and mix and match by adding any other product you like to it.
Liver health ½ cup broccoli ½ carrot½ apple ¼ fresh beetroot ½ lemon + peel	Pollution, sugar, highly processed foods all affect the liver. Added to that medications that are required may also hamper the liver. Taking the liver health a few times a week will flush the liver and keep it performing.

Hay-fever help (1) Whole orange + peel ½ lemon + peel ginger to taste (fresh) 1 teaspoon of quality honey **Hay-fever help (2)** 2 radish 1 orange + peel 1 apple 2 tablespoons of roast- ed lemon	Needing an anti-histamine? Here it is in a combination that has proven to be excellent. Use as a treatment or preven- tion.
Lower blood pressure ¼ beetroot ½ cucumber 1 apple ½ cup broccoli ½ carrot Pinch chilli (optional)	This combination is one that has been found to help with lowering blood pressure. Make sure you work with your doctor who will oversee any medica- tion you are taking.
Insomnia soother ½ cup lettuce 1 apple 1 egg	Insomnia soother utilises the nervine salts found within the lettuce and the settling magne- sium found in the apple

Urinary tract cleanse ½ cup raw cauliflower 1 apple 1 carrot ¼ cup of cucumber ½ cup of currents soaked in water 1 stick of celery	The urinary tract can struggle sometimes as it does a big job. This blend can be taken daily if you have a urinary tract weakness or taken a few times a week to cleanse.
Eye health 1 carrot ginger to taste 1 cup of berries (any) blueberries work well ½ cucumber unpeeled	The nutritional benefits for the eyes in this tonic are well researched particularly blue berries and carrot.
Fuel up tonic ginger to taste 1 apple ½ banana ¼ beetroot 2 stalks celery ½ cup sprouts (any) Almond milk	Feeling tired and run down? This is a fuel up blend that is excellent and many report they can feel it fuelling up the body as it goes down.

Illness recovery ½ avocado flesh 1 apple 2 leaves kale (lightly steamed) 1 roasted lemon Pinch chilli or black pepper	Often after illness we struggle to re-gain our energy. This blend can be taken daily until the energy builds and you are back on your feet.
Cold and flu recovery ¼ onion 1 roasted lemon 1 apple 2 tablespoons of honey Tip of teaspoon of chilli or black pepper 1 handful of parsley 1 handful of common mint	The immune system needs supporting and this combination draws on the best blend to provide results.

Cholesterol lowering

2 green beans

1 kiwi fruit (whole)

½ apple + peel

½ carrot ¼ beetroot

2 tablespoons of soaked rolled oats

Pinch of chilli (optional)

Pomegranate juice

Add almond, rice or oat milk for a smoothie or juice all the above adding the soaked oat into the juice.

This combination assists the gastrointestinal tract to take control of the bad guys when it comes to bad cholesterol. The blending of the oats aids the digestive system and the bowel to perform well and lower cholesterol. Fantastic and very popular blend bringing excellent results when combined with a sensible diet that also includes good hydration.

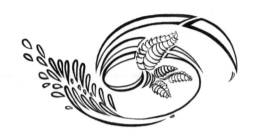

References

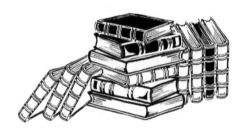

Adams, Ruth. 1982. The Complete Home Guide to All the Vztamins Larchmont Books, New York

Airola, Paavo, Ph.D., ND 1972 Cancer Causes, Prevention and Treatment, Health Plus Publishers. Arizona. USA

Airola, Paavo. Ph.D 1985 How to get well. Health Plus Publishers, Arizona USA –

Benowicz, Robert. J. 1983 Vitamins & You. Berkeley Books, New York m Buchman,

Dian Dincin. 1980 Feed for your face Duckworth London

Carper, Jean. 1988 The Food Pharmacy Simon & Schuster. London

Chao-liang, Chang.Et. A1. 1985 Vegetables as Medicine The Rams Skull Press Kuranda. Australia

Davies, Stephen, Dr &Stewan, Alan, Dr. 1987 Nutritional Medicine Pan Books London

Davis, Adelle. 1983 Let's Stay Healthy Unwin Publications. U SA

Dunne, Lavon. J. 1990 Nutrition Almanac 3rd Edition Mc-Graw—Hill Publications New York

English, Ruth. Lewis, Janine. 1992 Nutritional Values of Australian Foods Australian Government Publishing Services, Canberra.

Faelten, Sharon Et. A1. 1981. Complete Book of Minerals for Health. Rodale Press, USA

Gildroy. Ann. M.Sc. Nutrition. 1982 Vitamins and Your Health Unwin Publications.

Greer, Rita. 1982 Diets to help Multiple Sclerosis Thorsons Publications. London

Griffith, H. Winter. MD 1988. Complete Guide to Vitamins Minerals and Supplements

Fisher Books. Arizona. USA

Hall, Dorothy. 1989 The Natural Health Book Viking O'Neil Australia

Haas, Elsen. M, MD. 1992 Staying Healthy with Nutrition, Celestial Arts, Berkeley,

 California USA

Heinerman, John. 1988 Heinerman'sEncyclopedia of Fruits, Vegetables and Herbs, Parker Publishing. New York

Jensen, Bernard, Dr. 1988 Foods That Heal, Avery Publishing, New York

Jensen, Bernard. 1978 Nature Has a Remedy Jensen Publications, California, USA

Kadans, Joseph, Dr 1973 Encyclopedia of Fruits, Vegetables, Nuts and Seeds- Parker

Publishing New York

Kenton, Leslie & Susannah.1989 Raw Energy Arrow Books. London

Koch, Manfred. 1981. Laugh With Health Renaissance & New Age Creations. Australia

Lee, William. H. Ph.D 1982 The Book of Raw Fruit and Vegetable Juices and Drinks. Keats Publications. Connecticut. USA

Mervyn, Len. 1980. Minerals and Your Health Allen & Unwin London

Mervyn, Leonard. B.Sc., Ph.D., C.Chem., F.R.S.C. 1984 The Dictionary of Vitamzns :4; Lothian Publishers, Australia

Murray, Michael. N.D. Pizzorino 1990 Encyclopedia of Natural Medicine Mac Donald Opima, England

Murray, Michael. T. ND 1993 The Healing Power of Foods Prima Publishing. California. USA

Osiecki, Henry. 1990 Nutrients in Profile.Bioconcepts Publishing. Queensland Australia

Rubincarn, David & John. 1977. Diet with Vitamins A&W Publishers. New York

Sanders, Tom, BSC, Ph.DEt.Al 1997 *Foods That Harm Foods That Heal*. Readers Digest. Australia

Setright, Russell 1990 *Get Well An A-Z of Natural Medicine for Everyday Illness*. Atrand, NSW Australia

Tenney, Louise. 1991 *Louise Tenney's Nutritional Guide with Food Combining* Woodland Books. Utah. USA

Tisserand, Maggie. 1993 *Aromatherapy for Women*, Thorsons, London

Tisserand, Robert. Balacs, Tony. 1995 *Essential Oil Safety, A Guide for Health Care Professionals* Churchill Livingstone. USA

Valnet, Jean. MD. 1976 *Heal Yourself with Vegetables, Fruits and Grains*, Erbonia BOOKS

Van Stratten, Michael & Griggs Badoac. 1990 *Superfoods* Lothian Publishing, Melbourne

Walker, N.W. D.Sci. 1983 *Raw Vegetable Juices* Jove Books, USA

Worwood, Valerie Ann. 1990 *The Fragrant Pharmacy*, McMillan, London

Wright, Jonathan. V, M.D. 1990 Dr Wright's Guide to Healing with Nutrition. Keats Publishing, Connecticut, USA

http://www.healthline.com/natstandardcontent/gamma-linolenic-acid viewed 21/5/2014